FOUNDATIONS
OF PERINATAL GENETIC
COUNSELING

D1474317

Genetic Counseling in Practice
General Editor: Bonnie Baty

Foundations of Perinatal Genetic Counseling

A Guide for Counselors

Amber Mathiesen, MS, LCGC
Perinatal Genetic Counselor
Maternal and Fetal Medicine
University of Utah Health

Kali Roy, MS, LCGC
Perinatal Genetic Counselor
Maternal and Fetal Medicine
University of Utah Health

OXFORD
UNIVERSITY PRESS

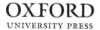

Oxford University Press is a department of the University of Oxford. It furthers the University's objective of excellence in research, scholarship, and education by publishing worldwide. Oxford is a registered trade mark of Oxford University Press in the UK and certain other countries.

Published in the United States of America by Oxford University Press
198 Madison Avenue, New York, NY 10016, United States of America.

Library of Congress Cataloging-in-Publication Data
Names: Mathiesen, Amber, author. | Roy, Kali, author.
Title: Foundations of perinatal genetic counseling : a guide for counselors /
Amber Mathiesen, Kali Roy.
Description: Oxford ; New York : Oxford University Press, [2018] |
Includes bibliographical references and index.
Identifiers: LCCN 2017041523 | ISBN 9780190681098 (pbk. : alk. paper)
Subjects: | MESH: Genetic Counseling | Prenatal Diagnosis
Classification: LCC RG628.3.A48 | NLM WQ 209

This material is not intended to be, and should not be considered, a substitute for medical or other professional advice. Treatment for the conditions described in this material is highly dependent on the individual circumstances. And, while this material is designed to offer accurate information with respect to the subject matter covered and to be current as of the time it was written, research and knowledge about medical and health issues is constantly evolving and dose schedules for medications are being revised continually, with new side effects recognized and accounted for regularly. Readers must therefore always check the product information and clinical procedures with the most up-to-date published product information and data sheets provided by the manufacturers and the most recent codes of conduct and safety regulation. The publisher and the authors make no representations or warranties to readers, express or implied, as to the accuracy or completeness of this material. Without limiting the foregoing, the publisher and the authors make no representations or warranties as to the accuracy or efficacy of the drug dosages mentioned in the material. The authors and the publisher do not accept, and expressly disclaim, any responsibility for any liability, loss or risk that may be claimed or incurred as a consequence of the use and/or application of any of the contents of this material.

9 8 7 6 5 4 3 2

Printed by Webcom, Inc., Canada

To our patients, who inspire us each and every day.

To our students, who gave us motivation and purpose for this endeavor.

To our teachers, who helped shape us.

None of whom we could have done this without.

CONTENTS

PREFACE

This book all started as an idea inspired by years of being genetic counselors and instructors of perinatal genetics. The inspiration was, "Why is there no single resource to learn the basic concepts of perinatal genetics?." The idea was "Why don't we write one ourselves?" After several conversations with other genetic counselors and educators, the idea became a dream: to make a resource that assisted in educating genetic counselors. The dream has now become a reality thanks to the support and collaboration of others.

Although this text is primarily designed for genetic counseling students, those teaching perinatal genetics, and the genetic counselor who is starting a perinatal position for the first time or after years in a different subspecialty, any health care provider interested in learning these concepts will benefit from the material presented in this book. Essential concepts and information needed to practice perinatal genetic counseling are discussed, including information about pregnancy, the components of a perinatal session, testing options and procedures, common indications, pregnancy management options, and ethical and unique situations encountered in the perinatal setting.

Foundations of Perinatal Genetic Counseling is just that: *the foundation* on which to build upon. Although many topics are reviewed, this book is meant to be a starting place and is not designed to be a standalone resource. Students and educators are encouraged to utilize the abundant resources and publications available as well as to take advantage of their individual experience and the collective knowledge of peers, other health care providers, and educators to complement what is learned in this text.

Ultimately, we couldn't be more excited to share this text for teaching and learning the foundations of perinatal genetics. We are confident that our ultimate goal of supporting the development of qualified, educated, and professional genetic counselors will be that much easier to achieve.

Amber Mathiesen, MS, LCGC
Kali Roy, MS, LCGC

ACKNOWLEDGMENTS

We would like to give a special thank-you to Bonnie Baty and to Oxford University Press for providing us with the opportunity to write this book. Without them, the idea for this book would have remained just that—an idea. We would also like to thank ARUP Laboratories for graciously providing us with several images for this text.

And, as always, thank you to our partners and families for always supporting and encouraging us to do what we love.

ABBREVIATIONS

AB	Abortion
AC	Abdominal circumference
ACOG	American Congress of Obstetricians and Gynecologists
ACMG	American College of Medical Genetics and Genomics
AFI	Amniotic fluid index
ADO	Allele dropout
AMA	Advanced maternal age
Amnio	Amniocentesis
APA	Advanced paternal age
ART	Assisted reproductive technologies
ASHG	American Society of Human Genetics
BMI	Body Mass index
BP	Blood pressure
BPD	Biparietal diameter
CBC	Complete blood count
cfDNA	Cell-free DNA
CMA	Chromosome microarray analysis
CRL	Crown–rump length
CVS	Chorionic villus sampling
ECT	Ectopic pregnancy

EDC/ EDD	Expected date of confinement/expected due date
DM	Diabetes mellitus
FL	Femur length
FOB	Father of the baby
G	Gravida
GA	Gestational age
GDM	Gestational diabetes mellitus
HbA1c	Hemoglobin A1c
HC	Head circumference
HTN	Hypertension
Hx	History
ICSI	Intracytoplasmic sperm injection
IOL	Induction of labor
ISPD	International Society of Prenatal Diagnosis
IUD	Intrauterine device
IUFD	Intrauterine fetal demise
IUGR	Intrauterine growth restriction
IUP	Intrauterine pregnancy
IVF	*In vitro* fertilization
L&D	Labor and delivery
LMP	Last menstrual period
MCA	Multiple congenital anomalies
MSS	Maternal serum screening
NICU	Newborn intensive care unit
NIPT/NIPS	Noninvasive prenatal testing or screening
NPV	Negative predictive value
NST	Non-stress test
NSGC	National Society of Genetic Counselors
NSVD	Normal spontaneous vaginal delivery
NT	Nuchal translucency
ONTD	Open neural tube defect
P	Para
PGD/PGS	Preimplantation genetic diagnosis or screening
PCR	Polymerase chain reaction
PPV	Positive predictive value

POC	Products of conception
RBC	Red blood cell
RPL	Recurrent pregnancy loss
SAB	Spontaneous abortion (miscarriage)
SB	Stillbirth
SMFM	Society for Maternal–Fetal Medicine
TOC	Transfer of care
TOP	Termination of pregnancy
VBAC	Vaginal birth after cesarean
VUS	Variant of uncertain significance

1

Pregnancy Basics

Perinatal genetic counselors have the privilege of working with people during one of the most significant experiences of their lives. Patients have many expectations, hopes, and dreams as well as fears, anxieties, and worries. Although a patient's provider (e.g., midwife, obstetrician, perinatologist) will manage her pregnancy and delivery, perinatal genetic counselors need to be aware of basic pregnancy concepts. This chapter provides background information on the components of routine prenatal care and testing as well as descriptions and instruction on how to document an obstetric history, establish a gestational age and due date, and use a pregnancy wheel and other similar tools.

Pregnancy Timeline and Dating

In addition to the patient wanting to know what to expect at certain points in pregnancy and when her baby will be arriving, knowing the timeline and having correct dating of a pregnancy is critically important for pregnancy management from the beginning to delivery. Accurate gestational dating is critical for the application and interpretation of certain tests (e.g., maternal serum screening) and for understanding risks from teratogen exposures, as well as obstetrical management of problems such as intrauterine growth restriction, preterm labor, and post-term pregnancy. This section will review the basic timeline of pregnancy as well as current guidelines and tools used for estimating due dates.

Pregnancies Are Counted in Weeks

Although many patients and the public in general use months to describe where they are in their pregnancy, in health care we use weeks and days as our measurement. For example, it is more accurate to describe a pregnant patient as being at 20 weeks than to say 5 months, which may be 20 weeks plus or minus a few weeks. The days of pregnancy are also included. For example, our patient who is in her 20th week may be 20 weeks and 0 days up to 20 weeks and 6 days. This is commonly written as 20w6d or 20 6/7 weeks.

Gestational Age Versus Embryonic Age

Gestational age and *embryonic age* (also referred to as *fetal age* or *development age*) are estimations of the age of the fetus in weeks. Typically in obstetric care, gestational age is utilized; however, embryonic age is important when considering embryonic development and timing of teratogenic exposures.

The use of gestational age is often confusing for patients and providers alike because it includes the 2 weeks before the patient's pregnancy was conceived. Gestational age is calculated from the patient's first day of her last menstrual period (LMP), whereas embryonic age starts at the date when the sperm fertilized the egg (also known as the date of conception and corresponds to the date of ovulation). Most women have 28-day menstrual cycles, counting from the first day of one menstrual period to the first day of the next menstrual period. Ovulation typically occurs at day 14 (2 weeks after a woman's LMP). Because of this, the gestational age is the embryonic age plus 2 weeks and the embryonic age is the gestational age minus 2 weeks. For example, a fetus that is at 12 weeks' gestation is 10 weeks by embryonic development.

Normal Pregnancy Timeline and Duration

Commonly used terms to describe what stage a woman is in regarding her pregnancy are *antepartum, intrapartum,* and *peripartum.* Antepartum is defined as the prenatal period or the time during pregnancy before birth. Intrapartum refers to the time during labor and delivery. Peripartum is the time during the last month of gestation and the first few months after delivery.

Based on gestational age, a pregnancy consists of 40w0d (280 days); however, pregnancy lengths between 38w0d and 42w0d are considered normal. Pregnancy consists of three trimesters. The *first trimester* is between 0w1d and 13w6d, the *second trimester* is 14w0d to 27w6d, and the *third trimester* is from 28w0d to the end of the pregnancy.

Pregnancy is also divided into three periods called the *germinal period, embryonic period,* and the *fetal period.* The germinal period begins at the time of conception with the formation of the *zygote,* the single cell formed from the union of the egg and sperm cells. The zygote begins actively dividing and moving down the fallopian tube to the uterus. The zygote eventually forms a structure called the *blastocyst,* which possesses an inner cell mass and an outer layer called the *trophoblast.* The inner cell mass will give rise to the fetus, and the trophoblast will become the placenta. Once the developing blastocyst reaches the uterus (typically 6–8 days after conception), it will begin to implant into the wall of the uterus. The germinal period ends when the blastocyst is fully implanted into uterine tissue (by the end of week 2 by embryonic age or end of week 4 by gestational age). Please see Figure 1.1.

The embryonic stage begins at the third week of development (5w0d gestation) and will continue until the end of the eighth week (end of 10 weeks gestation). The zygote is now termed the *embryo.* The most characteristic event occurring during this time is *gastrulation,* the process that establishes the three germ layers called the *ectoderm* (outer), *mesoderm* (middle), and *endoderm* (inner). Each germ layer will differentiate into different structures. Neurulation also takes place during this time, giving rise to the neural tube. This is a critical time for development as it is during the embryonic period when most of the organ systems are established (Moore, Persaud, 1998).

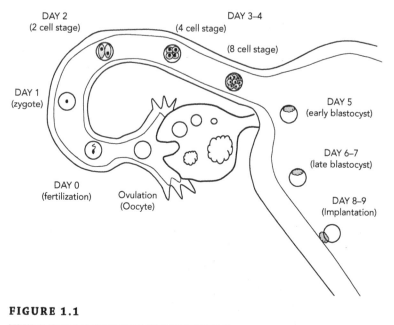

FIGURE 1.1

Ovulation to implantation.

The fetal period begins at 9 weeks embryonic age (11 weeks gestational age) to the end of the pregnancy. During the fetal period, the organs that formed during the embryonic period grow and differentiate into unique structures (organogenesis) (Moore, Persaud, 1998).

Methods for Dating

Pregnancy dating uses three methods: determining the first day of the patient's LMP or known conception date, ultrasound, and a physical exam. Often a combination of the three methods is used for proper dating and establishing the patient's expected due date (EDD).

Typically, determining the LMP is the first step in establishing an EDD. The date of the LMP corresponds to day 1 of the pregnancy. The EDD is 280 days from the LMP, or 40 weeks. It is important to note that women's menstrual cycles are of different length and can vary from 14 and 35 days. Ovulation can also be variable and may occur between 11 and 21 days after the LMP. The LMP method assumes ovulation and conception (fertilization) on day 14 and therefore does not account for irregularities in cycle length or variability in the timing of ovulation. Additionally, it has been found that only about one-half of women accurately recall their LMP date (Wegienka, Baird, 2005).

The date of conception can also be used when known. For example, many patients will utilize assisted reproductive technologies (ART) such as *in vitro* fertilization (IVF) or insemination. IVF involves manually combining eggs and sperm outside of the body and then later transferring an embryo into the uterus. (Please see Chapter 8 for more information on ART.) For patients undergoing IVF, the provider must consider the date of transfer into the uterus and the age of the embryo at that time. Typically, an embryo is transferred on day 3 or 5 after fertilization. The date of fertilization is considered week 2 of the pregnancy, and therefore transferring a 3-day embryo would correspond to 2w3d and a 5-day embryo would be a 2w5d. If the patient has completed an insemination, this would be considered the date of conception, and therefore the date of insemination is week 2 of the pregnancy.

Ultrasound is also used to date a pregnancy and is especially useful when the LMP is unknown or uncertain. The best time to use ultrasound for dating is in the first trimester (up to and including 13w6d). Dating from a first-trimester ultrasound is based on the mean of three separate measurements of the crown–rump length (CRL). The CRL is the measurement of the length of the embryo or fetus from the top of its head to bottom of its torso. Measurements of the CRL are more accurate the earlier in the first trimester that ultrasonography is performed. CRL measurements taken at or after 14w0d weeks (84 mm) decrease in accuracy. A later ultrasound (after 14w0d) can be used to date the pregnancy as well. In a later ultrasound, rather than using the CRL, other measurements including the biparietal diameter (BPD), head circumference (HC), femur length (FL), and abdominal circumference (AC) are used.

Pregnancies may also be dated with a physical exam, although this is the least accurate method and may be misleading due to factors including twins or other multiples, uterine tumors, or obesity. This method is not used to date the pregnancy if LMP or ultrasound is available.

Guidelines and Recommendations for Determining Dating

The American College of Obstetricians and Gynecologists, the American Institute of Ultrasound in Medicine, and the Society for Maternal–Fetal Medicine established a standardized approach for estimating gestational age and the anticipated due date (American College of Obstetricians and Gynecologists. 2014). This Committee Opinion recommends the following:

- Ultrasound measurement of the embryo or fetus in the first trimester (up to and including 13 6/7 weeks of gestation) is the most accurate method to establish or confirm gestational age.
- If pregnancy resulted from ART, the ART-derived gestational age should be used to assign the EDD. For instance, the EDD for a pregnancy resulting from IVF should be established using the age of the embryo and the date of transfer.
- As soon as data from the LMP, the first accurate ultrasound examination, or both are obtained, the gestational age and the EDD should be determined, discussed with the patient, and documented clearly in the medical record. Subsequent changes to the EDD should be reserved for rare circumstances, discussed with the patient, and documented clearly in the medical record.
- When determined from the methods outlined in this document for estimating the due date, gestational age at delivery represents the best obstetric estimate for the purpose of clinical care and should be recorded on the birth certificate. For the purposes of research and surveillance, the best obstetric estimate, rather than estimates based on the LMP alone, should be used as the measure for gestational age.

Based on these recommendations, one needs to know how to determine the "best obstetric estimate" by utilizing the data from both the LMP and the ultrasound. This statement outlines specific guidelines on how to combine the multiple data points and how to handle discrepancies between the different dating methods. Please see Table 1.1 for defined discrepancies. Box 1.1 gives some examples for practice.

- The first step is to document the LMP and date of conception (in cases of IVF or insemination).
- If the patient used ART, the ART-derived date should be used.
- If the patient conceived spontaneously, then comparison of the ultrasound and LMP dating is recommended.
- If there is a discrepancy between the ultrasound and LMP dating that deviates by more than the determined acceptable amount, then it is recommended to use the ultrasound dating.
- The acceptable discrepancy differs depending on the gestational age at which the ultrasound was completed.
- If the discrepancy is less than the acceptable amount, then it is recommended to use the LMP date.
- If a patient is unsure of her LMP date, the ultrasound date should be used.
- Last, once a gestational age is established subsequent deviations in later ultrasounds should not be used to alter the EDD or estimated gestational age.

Tools Available for Calculating Gestational Age

Multiple tools are available to assist with the determination of the due date and gestational age. Calculators exist on numerous websites (e.g., March of Dimes, American Pregnancy Association). These calculators allow input of various information including LMP and date of conception. From this information, a due date is calculated. Calculators have also been integrated into electronic medical record systems for easy reference. Cell phone calculator apps also exist.

TABLE 1.1 Guidelines for pregnancy dating when there are discrepancies

Gestational Age Range	Method of Measurement	Discrepancy Between Ultrasound Dating and LMP Dating that Supports Redating
≤8w6d	CRL	More than 5d
9w0d to 13w6d	CRL	More than 7d
14w0d to 15w6d	BPD, HC, AC, FL	More than 7d
16w0d wk to 21w6d	BPD, HC, AC, FL	More than 10d
22w0d to 27w6d	BPD, HC, AC, FL	More than 14d
28w0d and beyond	BPD, HC, AC, FL	More than 21d

BOX 1.1 Examples of Dating Recommendations

- A patient has an ultrasound at 8 weeks of pregnancy by LMP. The ultrasound suggests a 5-day discrepancy. Do you change the due date?
- A patient has an ultrasound at 8 weeks of pregnancy by LMP. The ultrasound suggests a 6-day discrepancy. Do you change the due date?
- A patient has an ultrasound at 8 weeks of pregnancy by LMP. The ultrasound suggests a 5-day discrepancy. She is later seen at 20 weeks by LMP, and there is an 11-day discrepancy. Do you change the due date?
- A patient has her first ultrasound at 20 weeks of pregnancy by LMP. The ultrasound suggests an 11-day discrepancy. Do you change the due date?

Answers: no, yes, no, yes

Perhaps the most widely used tool in a clinical setting is the pregnancy wheel. The pregnancy wheel consists of two circles. The outer circle is a year-long calendar. The inner circle is a count of a pregnancy from the LMP to 42 weeks of pregnancy. The inner circle is typically marked with key dates of the pregnancy such as LMP, probable date of conception, and EDD (40 weeks). The two circles can be rotated so that the LMP mark in the inner circle can fall on any date in the calendar. For example, if a patient reports an LMP of November 23, move the LMP mark to that date. The EDD mark on the inner circle would then line up with the EDD. For example, if the patient had an LMP of November 23, the EDD would be August 30. The probable date of conception would be December 7. In addition to using the LMP to get the EDD, the mark for the probable date of conception can be used if this is the date known. Figure 1.2 shows a pregnancy wheel.

The pregnancy wheel is useful for determining gestational age and EDD, but it is also helpful to easily and quickly calculate when the patient will reach certain points in her pregnancy. This

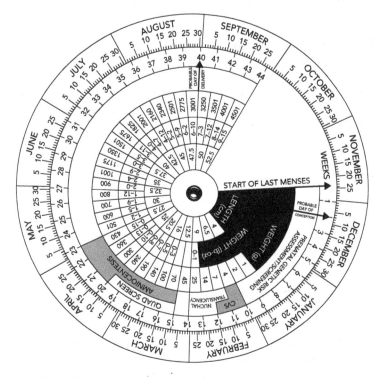

FIGURE 1.2

Pregnancy wheel.

is important when considering scheduling any follow-up testing or procedures. For example, when the EDD marked on the inner circle is at the EDD date of the patient, the genetic counselor can easily identify 16 weeks on the wheel and provide a date for a patient to return for an amniocentesis. It is important to note that pregnancy wheels do not take into account a leap year; during those years, the dating could be off by a day.

Pregnancy Care

As a health care provider working with pregnant patients, it is important to understand the basic principles of prenatal care and what the pregnant patient will experience during this time. This section will discuss basic prenatal care, common tests, and their significance.

Types of Prenatal Providers

Health care providers who care for pregnant patients include family practice doctors, obstetricians, certified nurse midwifes, and perinatologists (also known as maternal–fetal medicine specialists). Family practice doctors address the health care needs of whole families. Obstetricians and midwives specialize in working with pregnant patients. Perinatologists are further specialized to work with patients who have high-risk pregnancies. Perinatal genetic counselors typically work with perinatologists in high-risk pregnancy care, but they may see referrals from many other types of health care providers. These may include nurse practitioners, medical assistants, sonographers, radiologists, and reproductive endocrinologists.

Routine Prenatal Visits

The average pregnant patient is seen every 4 weeks from the beginning of pregnancy to the 28th week, every 2 weeks between weeks 28 and 36, and every week from week 36 to delivery. During each visit, the patient typically has her blood pressure, weight, and height checked as well as a screening to evaluate for glucose or protein in the urine. Fetal heart tones are also routinely evaluated. At the first appointment, the patient will have her blood drawn for the prenatal panel. Between 24 and 28 weeks, it is recommended for all patients to complete a screening test to determine if they have gestational diabetes. If the screen is abnormal, further testing is necessary. At 36 weeks, patients are screened for group B *streptococcus* and, if positive, given prophylactic administration of antibiotics to prevent transmission to the newborn during delivery.

Prenatal Panel

The prenatal panel is a group of blood tests completed at the beginning of the pregnancy or first prenatal appointment. The patient's provider will use this panel to evaluate for infections such as syphilis, chlamydia, and hepatitis B and C, as well as to see if the patient is immune to rubella or has been infected by the human immunodeficiency virus (HIV).

Complete Blood Count

A complete blood count (CBC) is a component of the prenatal panel. It is an evaluation that counts the number of white and red blood cells. This includes information on the red blood cell indices, which are the mean corpuscular volume (MCV), mean corpuscular hemoglobin (MCH), and mean corpuscular hemoglobin concentration (MCHC). Patients with low MCV (less than 80 fL) may have iron deficiency anemia or be carriers of a hemoglobinopathy. To evaluate for these, further testing is needed, including a serum iron ferritin level, hemoglobin electrophoresis, or molecular testing. (Please see Chapter 6 for further details for screening patients for hemoglobinopathies.)

Blood Type and Antibody Testing

The prenatal panel tests for blood type. A blood type is determined based on the type of antigens present on the surface of red blood cells. The blood group antigens are A, B, or O. Another common antigen complex is the Rh (CDE). Many other antigens exist, including Kell, Duffy, Kidd, and many others too numerous to list. Given that genes come in pairs, antigens do also. Thus a patient who is blood type A can be either A/A or A/O. Similarly, a person who is blood type B can be B/B or B/O. A person who is type O is O/O. Last, a person may be blood type A/B. Similarly with the Rh antigens, a person may have the RhD antigen present (+) or not (-). A person who is RhD(-) will be -/-, whereas a person who is RhD(+) may be +/+ or +/-. Approximately 15% of women with Caucasian ethnicity, 5–8% of African Americans, and 1–2% of Asians and Native Americans are RhD (-) (ACOG Practice Bulletin 75, 2006).

Documentation of the blood type is critical for proper management and prevention of alloimmunization (formation of antibodies). Although alloimmunization can result from many different antigens found on the red blood cell, RhD is the most common. If a patient with RhD(-) blood type is exposed to RhD (+) antigens, her body will produce antibodies against RhD. If a pregnant patient has any antibodies present, this may result in transplacental passage of the antibodies into the fetal circulation. This may lead to hemolytic disease of the fetus and neonate resulting in significant perinatal morbidity and mortality risks. Exposure typically happens during a pregnancy (caused by fetomaternal hemorrhage associated with delivery, trauma, spontaneous or induced abortion, ectopic pregnancy, or invasive obstetric procedures) or by blood transfusions. As a genetic counselor, you will see patients undergoing invasive procedures (e.g., amniocentesis and chorionic villi sampling). Documentation of the blood type is an absolute necessity prior to any patient undergoing either of these procedures. If a patient is RhD(-), then her provider will administer anti-D immune globulin prophylaxis (RhoGAM) to prevent alloimmunization.

The prenatal panel also evaluates patients for the presence of existing antibodies. If antibodies are present, then paternal, father of the baby (FOB) genotyping of the antigen of interest is recommended. Paternal testing will allow for accurate risk determination to the fetus by helping to predict the fetal antigen genotype without direct fetal testing unless necessary. For example, if you have a patient with RhD(–) blood type and anti-D antibodies are present, then paternal testing is indicated. If the FOB is tested and found to be RhD(–), the fetus is not at risk. If the FOB is Rh(+), he should be genotyped to determine if he is +/+ or +/–. If he is +/+, all pregnancies would be at risk. If he is +/–, then there is a 1 in 2 (50%) risk to each pregnancy and further testing could be pursued to determine the fetal genotype.

HbA1c for Diabetes

Maternal diabetes complicates approximately 2–3% of all pregnancies (National Center for Health Statistics, 1993). Maternal diabetes may be preexisting before pregnancy (pregestational diabetes) or have an onset during pregnancy (gestational diabetes mellitus). The majority (~90%) of cases of diabetes in pregnancy are gestational, which is associated with an increased risk for preeclampsia, cesarean delivery, and shoulder dystocia as well as fetal macrosomia, respiratory distress, and stillbirth. Pregnancies complicated by pregestational diabetes are at increased risk for congenital anomalies (e.g., open neural tube defects), miscarriage, stillbirth, and macrosomia. Measuring a patient's hemoglobin A1c (HbA1c) provides the cumulative effect of hyperglycemia over the past 2–3 months. The American Diabetes Association recommends an HbA1c goal of 6–6.5% and suggests that 6% may be optimal as pregnancy progresses (American Diabetes Association, 2016).

Fetal Imaging

Fetal imaging has many benefits including the determination of accurate gestational age, fetal number, placental location, fetal viability, and diagnosis of congenital anomalies. Ultrasounds may be performed in the first, second, or third trimester and are categorized as standard, limited, or specialized. Standard ultrasounds should be offered to all patients. A limited examination is performed when a specific question requires investigation or follow-up (e.g., vaginal bleeding, fetal position, etc.), and a specialized ultrasound is done when an anomaly is suspected and needs specialized evaluation, which may include fetal Doppler (allows for visualization of blood flow including in the umbilical cord, brain, and heart), biophysical profile (completed to measure fetal heart rate, muscle tone, movement, breathing, and amniotic fluid volume), amniotic fluid assessment, echocardiogram (targeted ultrasound of the fetal heart), or 3D ultrasound.

Traditionally, ultrasound has been offered only in the second trimester; however, first-trimester ultrasound (before 14 weeks) is increasingly performed. Ultrasound in the first trimester is typically done for determining the viability of the pregnancy and confirming gestational age as this is the most accurate for dating a pregnancy (Salomon et al., 2013). A first-trimester ultrasound may also be used for evaluation of a suspected ectopic pregnancy (when a fertilized egg implants outside of the uterus in the fallopian tube), vaginal bleeding, pelvic pain, maternal pelvic or adnexal masses or uterine anomalies, and suspected molar pregnancy. A specialized first-trimester ultrasound is also often used to evaluate risks of aneuploidy by measuring the nuchal translucency (fluid accumulation behind the neck), presence of the nasal bone, and ductus venosus waveform (refer to table 5.4). Additionally, in some centers it can be used to evaluate for severe fetal anomalies such as anencephaly.

The first-trimester ultrasound is also the best time to check for multiple gestations and, if identified, for chorionicity. Checking for chorionicity determines how many chorions are present. The *chorion* is the outer membrane that surrounds the *amnion*, the embryo and other membranes and entities in the womb. The amnion is the inner membrane. For example, twin pregnancies can be dichorionic and diamniotic (have two chorions and two amnions), monochorionic and diamniotic (have one chorion and two amnions), or monochorionic and monoamniotic (have one chorion and one amnion). It is important to determine this, given that monochorionic twins are at greater risks than are dichorionic twins, and this risk necessitates greater surveillance (Hack et al., 2008). Chorionicity also determines the likelihood that a multiple gestation originated from the same egg and sperm (monozygotic or identical) or from two separate eggs and sperms (dizygotic or fraternal). All monochorionic twins are monozygotic. Approximately 80–90% dichorionic twins are dizygotic; therefore although dizygosity is likely, it cannot be guaranteed.

A second-trimester ultrasound is ideally performed between 18 and 20 weeks gestation. Although indications for a second-trimester ultrasound may include many of the same as in the first trimester (e.g., evaluation for vaginal bleeding, dating, etc.), the second trimester is the ideal time to use ultrasound to evaluate fetal anatomy. Approximately 90% of infants with congenital anomalies are born to women with no risk factors (Long, Sprigg, 1998). Given this, it is recommended that all women be offered a second-trimester ultrasound that includes assessment of the fetal head (cerebellum, choroid plexus, cisterna magna, lateral ventricles, midline falx, cavum septi pellucidi), face (upper lip), neck, chest (heart), abdomen (stomach, kidneys, bladder, umbilical cord insertion, umbilical cord vessel number), spine, extremities, and sex (ACOG Practice Bulletin 101, 2009).

Third-trimester ultrasounds are typically performed for reevaluation of a fetal anomaly or progression of one. For example, the presence of mild ventriculomegaly identified in a second-trimester ultrasound may be followed to determine if it gets worse, better, or stays the same. This ultrasound may also be used to check fetal growth, fetal well-being, amniotic fluid levels, and fetal position for delivery.

Fetal magnetic resonance imaging (MRI) is another imaging modality offered to patients when there are specific anomalies suspected that need further assessment or to assist with facilitating management and decision-making on treatment when surgery or another intervention is being considered. Fetal MRI for screening is not used in the general population. Some common indications for fetal MRI include fetuses identified or suspected of having a central nervous system anomaly (e.g., agenesis of the corpus callosum, ventriculomegaly, holoprosencephaly), congenital diaphragmatic hernia, or myelomeningocele and in the evaluation of face and neck masses to determine if there is an airway obstruction. Fetal MRI has several advantages over prenatal ultrasound including that it is not as significantly limited by oligohydramnios (low amniotic fluid level), fetal positioning, maternal obesity, or shadowing from ossified bone. It also has superior contrast resolution and therefore can distinguish between fetal structures such as lung, liver, kidney, and bowel and thus allows for visualization of the entire fetus; this is better for evaluating fetuses with large or complex anomalies (Levine, 2001; Simon et al., 2000). MRI can be completed at 20–22 weeks' gestation as an adjunct to ultrasound; however, the third trimester is considered the optimal time.

Complicated Pregnancies

Patients with high-risk pregnancies may be seen by their provider more frequently. Although too numerous to note all, pregnancies can be complicated by multiple factors including multiple gestations, congenital anomalies, or maternal conditions such as seizures, gestational or preexisting diabetes, autoimmune disorders, thrombophilia, genetic syndromes (maternal phenylketonuria, achondroplasia, etc.), and cardiac disease. Pregnancies can also be complicated by current or a history of preterm labor, cervical insufficiency, and premature rupture of the membranes, preeclampsia, and chronic hypertension. Patients with these concerns may need additional support and specialty testing in their pregnancies. A referral to a perina-tologist is appropriate.

Documenting a Pregnancy History

A pregnancy history is a crucial part of documentation and may affect how a patient is counseled and managed. In this section, you will learn about the definition and significance of gravidity and parity, as well as how to calculate each value.

Gravida and Para

Gravidity and parity are important terms for gathering a woman's pregnancy history. *Gravida* is a term used to describe a woman who is pregnant. *Gravidity* is the total number of confirmed pregnancies a woman has had regardless of the outcome. Therefore, gravidity includes all miscarriages, terminations, ectopic pregnancies, stillbirths, and premature and live births. A woman who has never been pregnant is called a *nulligravida*, a woman who is or has been pregnant one time or who is in her first pregnancy is a *primigravida*, and a woman who has been pregnant more than once or is in at least her second pregnancy is a *multigravida*.

Para is defined as the number of times a woman has given birth to a pregnancy that is at least 20 weeks' gestation. This includes both stillbirths and live births. The term *nulliparous* is a woman who has never given birth, *primipara* is a woman who has had one child, and *multipara* is a woman who has had two or more births.

Calculating Gravidity and Parity (G's and P's)

Documentation of the pregnancy history is typically done in a shorthand system consisting of two sections. The first section, G, is a count for gravidity. This should include all confirmed current and past pregnancies. Each pregnancy is only counted one time, even if the pregnancy was a multiple gestation, such as twins or triplets. For example, a woman in her first pregnancy is written as G1 regardless if she is carrying a singleton or twin pregnancy.

The second section is written as P, which stands for parity. This section is expanded to include four points, *T*, term; *P*, preterm; *A*, abortion; and *L*, living children. All of these points get their own count. *Term* includes all full-term pregnancies: liveborn or stillborn at 37w0d gestation or after. *Preterm* stands for live birth or stillborn preterm deliveries between 20w0d and 36w6d. The *Abortion* section includes all spontaneous or induced abortions (miscarriages, terminations, and ectopic pregnancies) that are 19w6d or less. In these three points, all twin or other multiple pregnancies count as one. The last section, *Living Children*, includes all living children. In contrast to the preceding points, in this field each living child gets its own count. For example, a woman with one pregnancy of a singleton who delivered at full term would be written as G1P1001. A woman with a twin pregnancy who delivered at preterm, and both babies are living, is written as G1P0102. It is also important to note the living children section does not include any children who were adopted into the family. Please see Box 1.2 for a summary and Box 1.3 for some examples.

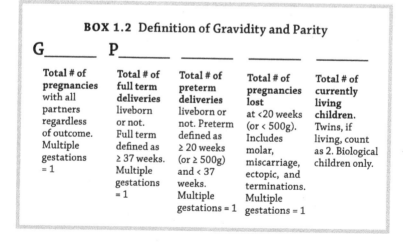

BOX 1.2 Definition of Gravidity and Parity

G_____   P_____   _____   _____   _____

Total # of pregnancies with all partners regardless of outcome. Multiple gestations = 1	Total # of full term deliveries liveborn or not. Full term defined as ≥ 37 weeks. Multiple gestations = 1	Total # of preterm deliveries liveborn or not. Preterm defined as ≥ 20 weeks (or ≥ 500g) and < 37 weeks. Multiple gestations = 1	Total # of pregnancies lost at <20 weeks (or < 500g). Includes molar, miscarriage, ectopic, and terminations. Multiple gestations = 1	Total # of currently living children. Twins, if living, count as 2. Biological children only.

BOX 1.3 Examples of G's and P's

- A woman with two 39-week deliveries, one 28-week twin delivery, one ectopic, all children living.

  (total # of pregnancies) = 4

  P: Term = 2, Preterm = 1, Abortions/miscarriages/ectopics = 1, Living children = 4

- A woman with two miscarriages, two term deliveries, currently pregnant, all children living, and one adopted child. (total # of pregnancies) = 5

  P: Term = 2, Preterm = 0, Abortions/miscarriages/ectopics = 2, Living children = 2

Conclusion

Every specialty of health care will have its own set of unique principles, vocabulary, and skills required for those entering and successfully practicing that specialty. Genetic counselors and other health care providers in the perinatal field will need to become familiar with pregnancy basics including the components of routine prenatal care, pregnancy duration and timing, and the stages of pregnancy. Becoming proficient in documenting an obstetric history by gravidity and parity, understanding how to establish gestational age and due dates, and being able to use a pregnancy wheel and other similar tools is essential in providing quality patient care. These basic principles will set the foundation for the practice of perinatal genetic counseling.

References

American College of Obstetricians and Gynecologists. Committee Opinion no. 611: Method for estimating due date. *Obstet Gynecol*. 2014;124:863–866.

American College of Obstetricians and Gynecologists. Practice Bulletin no. 101: Ultrasonography in pregnancy. *Obstet Gynecol.* 2009 Feb;113:451–461.

American College of Obstetricians and Gynecologists. Practice Bulletin no. 75: Management of alloimmunization during pregnancy. *Obstet Gynecol.* 2006 Aug;108:457–464.

American Diabetes Association. Management of diabetes in pregnancy. Sec.12. In Standards of Medical Care in Diabetes. *Diabetes Care.* 2016;39(Suppl. 1):S94–S98.

Hack KE, Derks JB, Elias SG. Increased perinatal mortality and morbidity in monochorionic versus dichorionic twin pregnancies: clinical implications of a large Dutch cohort study. *BJOG.* 2008;115(1):58–67.

Levine D. Ultrasound versus magnetic resonance imaging in fetal evaluation. *Top Magn Reson Imaging.* 2001;12:25–38.

Long G, Sprigg A. A comparative study of routine versus selective fetal anomaly ultrasound scanning. *J Med Screen.* 1998;5:6–10. (Level III)

Moore KL, Persaud TVN. *Before we are born: essentials of embryology and birth defects.* Philadelphia: WB Saunders, 1998.

National Center for Health Statistics: Prenatal care and pregnancies complicated by diabetes—U.S. reporting areas, 1989. *Morb Mort Wkly Rep.* 1993;42:119–122.

Salomon LJ, Alfirevic Z, Bilardo CM, Chalouhi GE, Ghi T, Kagan KO, et al. ISUOG practice guidelines: performance of first-trimester fetal ultrasound scan. *Ultrasound Obstet Gynecol.* 2013 Jan;41(1):102–113.

Simon EM, Goldstein RB, Coakley FV, Filly RA, Broderick KC, Musci TJ. Fast MR imaging of fetal CNS anomalies in utero. *AJNR Am J Neuroradiol.* 2000;21:1688–1698.

Ttrue12 (Own work). CC BY-SA 3.0 http://creativecommons.org/licenses/by-sa/3.0), via Wikimedia Commons from Wikimedia Commons.

Wegienka G, Baird DD. A comparison of recalled date of last menstrual period with prospectively recorded dates. *J Womens Health.* 2005;14:248–252.

2

The Perinatal Genetic Counseling Appointment and Family History

This chapter will outline the basic genetic counseling session as well as some considerations when taking a family history that are particularly relevant to the perinatal setting.

The Perinatal Genetic Counseling Session

The perinatal genetic counseling session has the same backbone as any other specialty session. However, there are aspects of the perinatal setting that are unique. In an ideal situation, the counseling would include time for each of the following sections; however, not all components will be relevant for every session, and some may involve two or more encounters to complete:

1. *Collect and review records and prepare for case.* Collecting records is an important first step in any genetic counseling session. The type of records collected will vary depending on the type of appointment and the reason for referral. In general, it is always important to gather records that indicate the patient's pregnancy history and outcomes, their care in the current pregnancy, any known family history already relayed to another provider, any testing already completed in this pregnancy (e.g., lab tests), and any ultrasound reports already

completed. When a patient has a referral for a family history of a genetic condition it is important to obtain records that confirm the diagnosis as well as the genetic mutation in the family member to allow for more accurate counseling and proper test ordering. This can lead to a genetic counselor discovering that the patient is not the ideal person in the family to test.

Preparing for the case allows the counselor to assess the referral from the patient's perspective and anticipate patient needs. Case preparation often starts with fact-gathering and can take time, especially when multiple references are needed. Fact-gathering is only the first half of the equation when it comes to preparing for a case. Taking the information that has been learned and creating a plan with the patient in mind allows the counselor to approach the upcoming appointment from a perspective that is most beneficial to the patient. It can also allow the counselor to determine which laboratories are the most appropriate for testing, how long the test will take to complete, and what the potential cost of a test might be and whether insurance will cover it. Case preparation is helpful in reducing the number of "surprise" questions that come up in a counseling session, as well as allowing the counselor to address questions that the patient did not know to ask.

2. *Contract with the patient, couple, or family.* Contracting allows the patient and the counselor to come to a mutual understanding about the reason for referral, what the appointment will entail, what will be discussed, and what to expect at each stage of the session. This allows both patient and counselor to make adjustments to their own expectations for the appointment prior to beginning. Some examples could include "tell me what you already understand about your appointment today" or "what information are you hoping to learn during your appointment?"

3. *Take pregnancy, medical, and family histories.* A family, medical, and pregnancy history is one of the most important steps in a perinatal genetic counseling session. A complete

evaluation of the family, medical, and pregnancy history allows the counselor to assess the risk for genetic conditions and birth defects, offer the most appropriate testing and make appropriate referrals. Taking a family history is commonly performed at the beginning of a genetic counseling session, but it can be done at any point, and it may be preferential to do so later depending on the patient or the feel and flow of the session. See the subsequent sections for a detailed description of obtaining a pregnancy and family history.

4. *Discuss the chance that a genetic condition has occurred in the current pregnancy or will occur in a future pregnancy.* This is often the heart of the perinatal genetic counseling session. Each session will have a different tone and topic depending on the reason for referral. An accurate discussion of this nature typically cannot be completed unless a thorough family, medical, and pregnancy history has been completed. Thorough research is often needed for these discussions, and research is often done prior to the appointment. This highlights the need for obtaining records prior to an appointment to ensure that you are prepared to speak appropriately about the concerns for this appointment.

5. *Explain the condition for which the pregnancy is at risk.* It is the counselor's role to be able to talk to patients about what a particular condition or ultrasound finding is in terms that are understandable to them. The goal is for them to be able to explain what the condition or the ultrasound finding is to another person. This can be challenging in a perinatal setting when the condition is unknown or the differential diagnosis is long and the topics discussed may be emotionally charged. Becoming educated in a particular condition or ultrasound finding takes time and a lot of research. Printed materials for the patient to reference at a later date are often a part of this discussion and can be helpful.

6. *Offer and discuss testing options.* A perinatal counselor will offer all available testing options to the patient as well as

discuss the benefits, limitations, and applicable risks of those options. This ensures that the patient has all the valid information needed to make an informed decision that is right for them with regard to their values. Testing options in the perinatal setting are sometimes limited by factors such as availability of fetal testing, gestational age, risks and benefits, availability of sample, and cost. Not all testing options will be available to all patients.

7. *Discuss test results and pregnancy management options and facilitate decision-making.* Once the test results are received, the counselor will need to talk with the patient about what they mean and do not mean. Once the test results are understood, then the counselor can present options for how to manage the current or future pregnancy based on those results. This should include the options of pregnancy termination, pregnancy continuation with either raising a child with special needs or making an adoption plan, and, in some cases, the availability of assisted reproductive technologies (ART) such as preimplantation genetic diagnosis or screening.

8. *Discuss implications for the future and for other family members.* Test results and ultrasound findings have an impact on the patient and the current pregnancy, but they could also have implications for subsequent pregnancies and other family members. Discussing these implications with the patient is important.

9. *Provide support resources.* Providing information regarding available support resources is part of what makes seeing a genetic counselor a unique experience compared to other providers. Support resources can include references, organized support groups, online forums and groups, contact information for other people who have had a similar experience, and the like.

10. *Make appropriate referrals.* It is often the genetic counselor who will make recommendations for who the patient should see to ensure the best care for their pregnancy.

11. *Documentation.* Documentation can take place in the format of clinic notes or letters. Clinic notes are typically a short description of the session including the reason for referral, what discussions occurred, and what decisions were made. Letters are often written to the referring provider or to the patient themselves. Letters are usually longer in length than a clinic note and provide more detail in terms discussions during the appointment, testing, test results if applicable, and recommendations for the pregnancy. Much has been written about how to write a proper patient or provider letter, thus we defer to those references for a full description.

Obtaining a Pregnancy History

Collecting and documenting the patient's pregnancy history is a typical component of any perinatal genetic counseling session. The provider should document how many pregnancies the patient has had, regardless of the outcome (e.g., delivered, miscarriage, ectopic, etc.), and the order in which pregnancies took place. It is helpful to include information on fetal sex (if known), alive or deceased, and any complications known (e.g., diagnosis of Down syndrome). People may have multiple partners in their lives, and therefore it should be noted if all pregnancies are with the same or a different partner. The patient's current partner should be asked if he has children or any pregnancies from a different union.

If a patient currently pregnant, the genetic counselor should inquire about any pregnancy complications such as bleeding, severe cramping, infections, or fevers of 100.4°F or higher. Bleeding in pregnancy is a common finding that can impact the performance of certain testing (e.g., maternal serum screen) or signify a miscarriage. Cramping is also normal, but if it is severe it may suggest a pregnancy loss or other complication and the patient may benefit from further evaluation or referral. Patients with high fevers early in the pregnancy are at increased risk for open neural tube defects, and testing should be offered. Medication use (including prenatal vitamins and when they started) and other exposures of concern (e.g., drugs, alcohol, cigarettes) should be noted. This allows for documentation of any teratogenic exposures that need to be addressed.

The perinatal counselor should determine the method of conception (i.e., if the pregnancy was achieved spontaneously or by *in vitro* fertilization [IVF]). If a patient achieved a pregnancy with the use of IVF, then one should ask if her own eggs were used and if it was a fresh or frozen cycle. If the patient used a donor egg, the age of the donor when eggs were collected is needed as this changes the risk of aneuploidy. Similarly, if the patient achieved a pregnancy from a frozen IVF cycle, the age of the patient at the time the eggs were retrieved should be documented. If a sperm donor was used, this is also important to note.

Last, any health complications or chronic conditions the patient has should be documented such as a personal history of diabetes, seizure disorder, cardiac disease, autoimmune disorder, or history of deep vein thrombosis, to name a few.

Obtaining a Family History

A lot has been written on the art and method of obtaining a family history. The family history is a fundamental part of a genetic counseling session. It is well accepted that a genetic counselor must be an expert at obtaining and documenting a quality family history. When complete, a pedigree can provide a quick visual reference for family relationships and any conditions, both Mendelian and multifactorial, present in a family, as well as help the counselor provide risk assessment (Bendure, 2006; Bennett, 2012). The process of taking a family history can aid in the development of rapport with the patient, couple, or family as it is often one of the first things completed in a genetic counseling session. The act of taking a family history can allow a counselor to establish a dialogue, establish trust from the patient, and learn about the family dynamics, and aid the counselor in determining anxiety levels (Bennett, 2012).

A three-generation pedigree is considered standard and is usually sufficient, although some circumstances may require a larger pedigree (ACOG, 2011). A perinatal family history is obtained just as it is in any other clinical setting, and standard symbols and nomenclature are used (Bennett, 2008). See Figure 2.1 for particularly relevant symbols in the perinatal setting. Please refer to the publication *Standardized Human Pedigree Nomenclature: Update and Assessment of the Recommendations* of the National Society of Genetic Counselors for complete pedigree nomenclature information (Bennett, 2008).

Interpreting a Family History

Learning to interpret a family history is a process that takes time and practice. There are certain things to look for in a family history that every genetic counselor, regardless of the specialty, must know. However, there are particular family history indications that are more relevant in the perinatal setting.

Mendelian Conditions

Interpreting family history of a single-gene condition is a relatively simple task. If the patient knows the name of the condition, research can be completed ahead of the appointment to determine the inheritance pattern (Bennett, 2008; ACOG, 2011). Often, a patient will attend a perinatal genetic counseling session for a different reason and bring up the family history of a genetic condition during the family history taking. A counselor can then ask about who else in the family is affected, how the diagnosis was made, who in the family has other signs or symptoms, and other details to be able to provide risk assessment to the patient (ACOG, 2011).

Pregnancy (P)	Male	Female	Unknown	Used to identify an ongoing pregnancy.
	☐ P	◯ P	◇ P	

Stillbirth (SB)	Male		Female	Stillbirth is pregnancy loss after 20 weeks gestation. Include gestational age and test results if known.
	◻ SB 25 wk		● SB 47, XX, +21	

Pregnancy loss	Spontaneous abortion (SAB)	Termination of pregnancy (TOP)	Ectopic pregnancy (ECT)	Include gestational age and test results if known.
	△ 12 wk	▲ 12 wk 45, X	◁ ECT	

Multiple gestation	Monozygotic	Dzygotic	Unknown	Trizygotic	A horizontal line between each individual's line indicates monozygosity. If unknown a question mark can be used.
			?		

Adoption	Adopted in to family	Adopted out to family	By Relative	Dashed line represents an individual adopted in the family (not biologically related). A solid line indicates an individual adopted out (biologically related).

Gamete donor	Ovum donor		Sperm donor	A woman carrying a pregnancy conceived with an ovum or sperm donation.
	D		D	
	P		P	

Surrogate	Surrogate only		Surrogate ovum donor	If the surrogate used the couples gametes she is a surrogate only. A surrogate may also be the ovum donor.
	S		D	
	P			

FIGURE 2.1

Common pedigree symbols in the perinatal setting.

Multifactorial Conditions

Multifactorial conditions are present in many patients' family histories. Multifactorial conditions are conditions that likely have a genetic component combined with other nongenetic factors that influence the expression of that condition (e.g., mental health conditions, diabetes, and adult-onset heart disease) (Bennett,

2012). A perinatal counselor should be able to talk to a patient about a multifactorial condition and provide risk assessment for that condition even though it is not inherited in a Mendelian pattern.

Consanguinity

Consanguinity is the term used for two partners who are descended from one ancestor; for example, first cousins. While this situation may seem theoretical, there are many couples who come for genetic counseling and who are related by blood. Knowing whether a couple is related by blood helps in perinatal risk assessment for recessive genetic conditions, birth defects, and adverse pregnancy outcomes (ACOG, 2011; Bennett, 2002). It is essential that every couple be asked if they are related by blood.

Birth Defects

In a perinatal family history we always ask about family history of birth defects (ACOG, 2011). Birth defects are most often isolated, but they can recur in families. Determining who in the family was born with a structural defect and how that person is related to the patient and/or the fetus will provide information for risk assessment. Birth defects can also lead a counselor down the path of suspecting an undiagnosed genetic condition in a family. Birth defects can also provide an explanation for an infant death.

Intellectual Disability and Autism

Intellectual disability and autism can be isolated conditions, multifactorial, or part of a genetic syndrome. A perinatal counselor should ask all patients about both of these conditions (ACOG, 2011). Autism and intellectual disability are common symptoms of genetic conditions and can thus be more than simply a diagnosis of "autism" or "intellectual disability." The counselor should ask follow-up questions regarding any person with a general description like autism or intellectual disability to determine if she has any additional characteristics that might indicate an underlying genetic condition, such as unique facial features different from family background, other symptoms, and any testing that might have been performed. Any person with a family history of autism or intellectual disability of unknown etiology or underlying diagnosis should be offered the option of fragile-X testing (ACOG, 2017; ACOG, 2006; Sherman, 2005). Fragile-X is the most common inherited form of intellectual disability (Lyons et al., 2015).

Pregnancy Loss and Infertility

Infertility is the inability to achieve a pregnancy within 12 months of unprotected intercourse (Practice Committee ASRM, 2013). There are many causes of infertility that include both male and female factors. The topic of infertility will be discussed in greater detail in Chapter 5. However, it is important for a perinatal genetic counselor to understand that there are genetic conditions that can cause infertility. A perinatal genetic counselor must know how to take a family history to elicit the greatest amount of information regarding these situations as well as interpret a family history where infertility is present.

Recurrent pregnancy loss is distinctly different from infertility, with the definition being two or more failed clinically recognized pregnancies (ACOG, 2011; Practice Committee ASRM, 2013). The pregnancy losses do not need to be consecutive. There are many causes of pregnancy loss, with only a small portion of those being related to genetics or genetic conditions. A perinatal genetic counselor must be able to speak to a patient regarding recurrent pregnancy loss even if the losses are unlikely to be related to genetic conditions. A perinatal genetic counselor must be able to recognize when recurrent pregnancy loss has occurred, take an accurate family history, know what follow-up questions to ask, and understand what testing options are available and recommended. It is important to distinguish among a spontaneous pregnancy loss (miscarriage), an ectopic pregnancy, and an elective termination of a pregnancy (Bennett, 2012). It is also important to note the gestational age of the fetus at the time of the demise. These can all impact risk assessment and proper counseling regarding testing options (Bennett, 2012). Male relatives whose partners (who are not blood related) have had pregnancy losses are important to the family history as pregnancy losses and many patients do not tend to report these losses. This information is important because the fetus that miscarried is still a blood relative and shares genetic ancestry with the patient.

Unknown Etiologies

There are many situations in a perinatal setting where a patient is unsure of the cause of a miscarriage, stillbirth, death, intellectual disability, or the like in a family member. It is important for the genetic counselor to acknowledge that the information is unknown and provide information about why it may or may not be important to obtain records for proper risk assessment. The only way a perinatal genetic counselor can be certain of a diagnosis or etiology is when records are obtained and reviewed for confirmation. It is also common for an etiology to be unknown after appropriate medical workup. When this occurs, a perinatal genetic counselor must be able to perform a general risk assessment with the information that is known. Sometimes there are evaluation guidelines when a diagnosis or an etiology is not known, such as in the fragile-X screening mentioned previously.

Accuracy

Inaccuracies in family histories are a certainty in any genetic counseling session. Patients often misremember names of diagnoses, ages of onset, or symptoms in a relative. Sometimes patients do not understand that there can be varying causes of the same condition. Patients may also misreport how a person is related to them (e.g., a first cousin once removed instead of a second cousin) or assume that a condition comes from a non-blood relative's side of the family and not theirs. In addition, records are not always available for confirmation, and patients may not have contact with certain pertinent relatives. Therefore, family history should always be interpreted with this in mind.

Other Conditions (Referrals)

It is not uncommon for a perinatal genetic counselor to be asked by a patient to test for or evaluate a patient (and not the pregnancy specifically) for a genetic condition that is in the family. A patient may become interested in knowing his or her risk for a specific condition in the family after the counselor takes a complete family history. While perinatal genetic counselors are educated in all types of genetic conditions, it is usually not appropriate to test a patient for a condition that will have no impact on the pregnancy or pregnancy management. Referrals are a large part of a perinatal genetic counselor's role. The counselor must know when it is most appropriate to refer a patient to another genetic counselor or type of provider (ACOG, 2011). For example, a pregnant patient comes in for prenatal screening and, during the family history, reports that her sister was recently diagnosed with breast cancer and found to carry a *BRCA1* mutation. The patient asks if you can just test her for the mutation. In this case, the genetic counselor has the ability to order *BRCA1* testing on the patient, but the most appropriate course of action is to refer the patient to a genetic counselor who specializes in cancer or a family cancer assessment clinic.

Unique Situations in the Perinatal Family History

In the perinatal setting there may be some unique situations that arise when taking a family history that may impact the risk assessment and interpretation of the pedigree.

Gamete Donation

Couples, of the same or opposite sex, can use gamete donors to conceive a pregnancy. Gamete donation can take place in the form of egg or sperm donation and is used for various reasons. It is important to take the family and medical history of the donor as well as of the intended parents, when applicable. There are various requirements evaluations of an egg or a sperm donor during the process of donation. Currently, guidelines for minimal evaluation requirements are set by the American Society of Reproductive Medicine (ASRM, 2012), but individual gamete donors can vary in their actual requirements. Many egg and sperm donors will have a family history questionnaire that is available to the couple utilizing the gamete. Some gamete donors will complete various genetic testing, such as carrier screening for any number of conditions and chromosome karyotype. It is important to obtain records for any of the evaluations that have been completed. If the gamete donation is from a friend or a relative, it is acceptable to ask the couple to provide any family history or testing information that is known. If the gamete donor is a relative, the counselor will want to note the relationship to the pregnant patient (e.g., sister, cousin).

Gathering any information on the gamete donor is important as it can change the risk assessment for a pregnancy. When a woman uses a donated egg, the age and family history of the donor impacts the risk for many genetic conditions. For example, if a woman who is 40 uses an egg donor who was 24 at the age of donation, the risk for chromosomal aneuploidy is that of a 24-year-old and not a 40-year-old. It might also be important to record family and medical history from both females, the genetic contributing mother and the gestational mother. A woman carrying a fetus who does not have her own genetic contribution still has an impact on the pregnancy itself and perhaps on the epigenetics of the developing fetus (Best, Carey, 2013).

Same-Sex Couples

Couples who are of the same sex often use ART to have children. When encountering a female same-sex couple, it is important to determine who is carrying the pregnancy and whether that is the person whose eggs were used for the conception. It is important to make sure the relationship lines are accurate (see Figure 2.1). Many female couples will use an intrauterine insemination from a sperm donor. Donor sperm may be from a sperm bank or from a person the couple knows, such as a friend or relative. When recording a family history in this situation, the counselor would want to ask about the family history of the sperm donor, if known. As with an opposite-sex couple, it is important to obtain records for any testing that has been completed. In these cases, it is not essential to collect family history information from the female partner not carrying the pregnancy or contributing her egg. However, many counselors will ask about her family in order to build rapport and be inclusive of the couple as a whole.

Some female couples elect to use an egg from one partner and implant the fertilized embryo in the other partner in order to share the pregnancy experience. In this case, it is important to record a family history from both female partners: the genetic contributing mother and the gestational mother. As with opposite-sex couples, the family and medical history of the egg donor will impact the risk assessment. Gathering information on the sperm donor follows the same process described earlier. As can be seen, this can quickly become a more complicated pedigree to draw.

Male same-sex couples may use a surrogate to carry a pregnancy in which one of the men is the biological father of the fetus (see the next section on surrogacy).

Surrogacy

Surrogacy is another situation that can arise in the perinatal pedigree. *Surrogacy* is when a female carries a fetus for another couple. This can be done with the use of the surrogate's own egg and the male partner's sperm, in which she becomes the surrogate and the egg donor. Another form is called *gestational surrogacy*, where a couple undergoes IVF using the intended mother's own egg (or an egg donor) and sperm from the intended father and the resulting embryo is subsequently transferred to a surrogate female who has no genetic connection to the embryo (ACOG, 2016). Those who are the intended parents—and ultimately take the baby home after birth—are called the *recipients*.

Surrogacy is often used for same-sex male couples as well as for opposite-sex couples for various medical reasons. For the same reason listed previously, it is important to gather information about the genetic egg and sperm donors for accurate risk assessment. In these situations, it is not uncommon to have the intended parents of the fetus attend the appointment, and they are typically the ones making the decisions regarding the pregnancy, including which, if any, testing they wish to pursue.

Adoption

Adoption is a situation that arises very often in any situation where a family history is taken. Sometimes it is a patient or a patient's partner who is adopted, and they can sometimes have little to no information about their biological parents and family history. This can sometimes be the source of much anxiety for future parents and may often be the reason that a patient or couple has sought genetic counseling. It is important to remember that everyone has "parents," and not having information about one's biological parents is not something to be ashamed of. We do not automatically treat those with limited or no family history information as "high risk"; rather, we assume them to be at a risk level comparable to the general population.

Adoption can come in the form of a family having a child who has been adopted into the family or a child who was adopted out of the family. These situations are unique from each other and should be marked on the pedigree accurately (see Figure 2.1). Determining the reason for adoption in or out of the family can help with risk assessment. For example, if the couple adopted out a baby who had Down syndrome, then their risk for a subsequent pregnancy with an aneuploidy increases as opposed to a couple who adopted out a baby because they were not ready to be parents at that time.

Ethnicity

Asking about a couple's ethnic background is important in a perinatal setting because it allows the counselor to provide information about the risk of being a carrier of certain recessive genetic conditions or the risk for particular multifactorial conditions, as well as to offer ethnicity-based testing recommended by guidelines (ACOG, 2017). Certain tests can also have different sensitivity and specificity depending on the patient's ethnicity, which is important to communicate. Sometimes a patient does not know their ethnicity. At other times, patients may interpret ethnicity as the state or country where they were born as opposed to their biological ancestry. A genetic counselor may need to clarify.

Conclusion

The ability to effectively conduct a perinatal genetic counseling session is important to overall quality of care. Some components of a perinatal genetic counseling session are similar to other subspecialties, such as case preparation, contracting, family history-taking, and explaining inheritance. Other components have nuances specific to the perinatal setting, such as taking a pregnancy history, risk assessment in pregnancy, and discussing the testing options available during pregnancy. In addition, there are unique situations that are important to understand as they may impact the structure and type of information provided during a session. An understanding of both the key elements of a perinatal counseling session and the unique situations that can affect these elements is a crucial foundation of perinatal genetic counseling.

References

American College of Obstetricians and Gynecologists Committee on Genetics. ACOG committee opinion no. 691: Carrier Screening for Genetic Conditions. Obstet Gynecol. 2017 March;129:41–55.

American College of Obstetricians and Gynecologists Committee on Genetics. Committee Opinion no. 478: family history as a risk assessment tool. *Obstet Gynecol.* 2011 Mar;117(3):747–750.

American College of Obstetricians and Gynecologists' Committee on Ethics, Ryan GL. ACOG Committee Opinion no. 660: family building through gestational surrogacy. *Obstet Gynecol.* 2016 Mar;127(3):e97–e103.

Bendure WB, Mulvihill JJ. Perform a gene test on every patient: the medical family history revisited. *J Okla State Med Assoc.* 2006 Feb;99(2):78–83.

Bennett RL, French KS, Resta RG, Doyle DL. Standardized human pedigree nomenclature: update and assessment of the recommendations of the National Society of Genetic Counselors. *J Genet Couns.* 2008 Oct;17(5):424–433.

Bennett RL, Motulsky AG, Bittles A, Hudgins L, Uhrich S, Doyle DL, et al. Genetic counseling and screening of consanguineous couples and their offspring: recommendations of the National Society of Genetic Counselors. *J Genet Couns.* 2002 Apr;11(2):97–119.

Bennett RL. The family medical history as a tool in preconception consultation. *J Community Genet.* 2012 Jul;3(3):175–183.

Best JD, Carey N. The epigenetics of normal pregnancy. *Obstet Med.* 2013;6(1):3–7.

Practice Committee of American Society for Reproductive Medicine. Definitions of infertility and recurrent pregnancy loss: a committee opinion. *Fertil Steril.* 2013 Jan;99(1):63.

Lyons JI, Kerr GR, Mueller PW. Fragile X syndrome: scientific background and screening technologies. *J Mol Diagn.* 2015 Sep;17(5):463–471.

Sherman S, Pletcher B, Driscoll D. ACMGC Practice Guideline Fragile X syndrome: diagnostic and carrier testing. *Med Gen.* 2005 Oct;7(8):584–587.

3

Prenatal Screening

Prenatal screening is a large component of a perinatal genetic counselor's job, whether it is in terms of discussing and offering screening to a patient, interpreting and providing results, or managing referrals based on abnormal results.

Evaluation of a Screen

Before discussing the details of the various prenatal screening options, it is important to understand some basic concepts of screening tests and how they are evaluated. This includes learning the definitions and calculations of several key concepts.

A screening test, by medical definition, is "the systematic application of a test or inquiry, to identify individuals at sufficient risk of a specific disorder to benefit from further investigation or direct preventive action, among persons who have not sought medical attention on account of symptoms of that disorder" (Wald, 2008). It is important to note the use of the word "inquiry" in the definition. Not all screening takes place in the form of a laboratory test on a bodily fluid (i.e., blood, urine, sweat, etc.). An inquiry in the form of a family history is equally valuable as a screening test (Guttmacher, 2004) and is often the easiest to obtain, highly informative, and the most cost-effective method for "identifying individuals at sufficient risk" to benefit from further investigation.

It is extremely important to note that screening tests do not diagnose a patient or a fetus with a condition and only serve to identify those at increased risk for a condition. In order for a screen to be effective, the risk of misclassification should be tolerably low. A screening test result is usually either positive (high risk) or negative (low risk), and these results can either be correct or incorrect, meaning the individual either does or does not have the condition they are being tested for. In the perinatal setting, a patient can complete laboratory test screening for the fetus or screening on themselves for various conditions even if the patient or the fetus does not have any signs or symptoms of that condition. The American College of Obstetricians and Gynecologists (ACOG) recommends that prenatal screening be offered to all pregnant patients (ACOG, 2016).

To understand screening, it is important to understand the common nomenclature that is used to evaluate how well a particular screen works. There are three main criteria used to determine the usefulness of a genetic screening test: analytic validity, clinical validity, and clinical utility. *Analytic validity* is how accurately the test measures the genotype of interest. *Clinical validity* is how well the test results correlate with what is seen clinically (phenotype). *Clinical utility* is the measure of how useful a test is in determining or changing the clinical management of the patient completing the test (Grosse, 2010). A genetic counselor will take all of these into consideration when offering a genetic screen to someone.

Being able to determine, understand, and explain the clinical validity of a screening test is an essential part of the evaluation of a screening test. Most patients will want to know how "accurate" a test is before deciding if it is the right course of action for them. This is usually the layman's term for the clinical validity of a test. Clinical validity is further broken down into specific measurements that help determine "accuracy": sensitivity, specificity, positive predictive value, and negative predictive value. Each component will be discussed in detail because these can be confusing, especially considering that alternative terms are used for the same measurements.

Sensitivity

Sensitivity is the proportion of affected individuals who have a positive test result. The synonyms for sensitivity are *detection rate* and *true-positive rate*. Detection rate is often used when speaking to a patient about the ability of a test to "detect" a certain condition in themselves or their fetus. In other words, the sensitivity of a test is how well the test correctly identifies those who have a condition with a positive test result (Lalkhen, 2008; Grosse, 2010; Loong, 2003; Wald, 2008). A screening test with higher sensitivity will identify more individuals who have a condition than will a screening test with a lower sensitivity. For example, a test with 90% sensitivity will detect 90% of patients who have the condition. Screening tests will be able to identify most people with a condition but not all.

Specificity

Specificity is the proportion of unaffected individuals who have negative results. The synonym for specificity is the *true-negative rate*. This measures the percentage of individuals who do not have a condition and who are correctly given a negative result (Lalkhen, 2008; Groose, 2010; Loong, 2003; Wald, 2008). The opposite of this is the *false-positive rate* or the rate at which those who do not have a condition will be misidentified. This term is often better understood by the average patient. This is because the focus is on that group of individuals who will be offered further testing and evaluation unnecessarily (Wald, 2008). In general, the higher the specificity of a test is the less likely you are to give someone a positive result when that individual does not have a condition.

It is common to see sensitivity and specificity explained by way of a table. A laboratory will use a table like this to determine the sensitivity and specificity of its particular test. Sensitivity and specificity are rates or a percentage and are calculated by dividing the number of true positives by the total number of positives for sensitivity and dividing the number of true negatives by the total number of negatives for specificity. See Table 3.1.

TABLE 3.1 Calculating sensitivity and specificity

	Condition Status	
Test result	Has the Condition (Affected)	Does Not Have the Condition (Not Affected)
Positive	A	B
Negative	C	D

(Lalkhen, 2008)

A = the number of people who have the condition and have a positive test result (correctly identified)
A = true positive
B = the number of people who do not have the condition but still got a positive test result (incorrectly identified)
B = false positive
C = the number of people who have the condition but got a negative test result (incorrectly identified)
C = false negative
D = the number of people who do not have the condition and got a negative test result (correctly identified)
D = true negative
A/A + C = sensitivity
D/B + D = specificity

There is a delicate balance that must occur when evaluating a test based on these measurements. It would seem that having a test that has high sensitivity and high specificity would be ideal. A "perfect" test would identify all of the patients who have a condition and would never be positive in a patient who does not have a condition. However, sensitivity can only increase at the expense of specificity and vice versa because they are inversely related. This is because the sensitivity and specificity of a test are determined by the cutoff point used to determine who is "positive" versus who is "negative." There will always be some overlap, even if it is very small, in the values measured by the

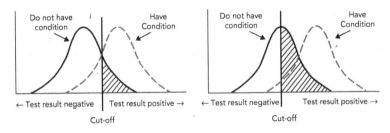

FIGURE 3.1

How cutoff affects test performance.

test of those who have a condition and those who do not (remember that screening does not have the ability to diagnose someone with a condition). If the cutoff point is moved so that it captures more of those with a condition, it will inherently also capture more of those without a condition (increase the false-positive rate). See Figure 3.1.

A clinician or a genetic counselor can use the sensitivity and the specificity of a particular test to compare to other types of tests or to determine if the test is useful.

Positive Predictive Value

Positive predictive value (PPV) refers to the likelihood that once a positive result is received by an individual, it will be a correct result. This can also be called the *odds of being affected given a positive result* (OAPR) (Lalkhen, 2008; Groose, 2010; Loong, 2003; Wald, 2008). Another way to view the PPV: out of all the positive results, how many belonged to individuals who actually had a condition? An individual's PPV can be calculated using Bayesian analysis. Refer to Table 3.1, where A/A + B = PPV.

Negative Predictive Value

Negative predictive value (NPV) is the opposite of PPV. It is the likelihood that a person with a negative result truly does not have the condition being tested for (Lalkhen, 2008; Groose, 2010; Loong, 2003; Wald, 2008). As in the preceding section: out of all the negative results, how many individuals truly do not have a condition? Refer to Table 3.1, where D/C + D = NPV.

PPV and NPV are evaluations made after a test has been completed and are not properties of the test itself. These are sometimes called *post-test probabilities*. The unique thing about PPV and NPV is that they are impacted by the sensitivity and specificity but can change when the prevalence of a condition changes. *Prevalence* is the proportion of the population who has a condition. When a condition is rare (and sensitivity and specificity of a test remain the same), the PPV will decrease. This is because when a condition is rare, it is unlikely that the person we are testing will have that condition and so a negative result is much more likely to be correct. In other words, you have to test a whole lot of people who are not very likely to have a condition in order to find that one individual who does. This becomes important for a perinatal genetic counselor when a prenatal screening test result returns with a positive result. The patient will want to know what the chances are that she is in the category of true positive (the condition is present) or the chance that her result is a false positive (the condition is not present, but we frightened her). Due to this, a screening test with really high sensitivity and specificity can have a very low PPV. For example: if Condition X has a prevalence of 1 in 1,000 in the population, then in a population of 10,000 pregnancies 10 of those pregnancies will actually have Condition X and 9,990 will not. Using the formula from Table 3.1, if all of those women screen their pregnancies for Condition X using a test with 99% sensitivity and 99% specificity, then we would expect to have 10 true-positive test results and 20 false-positive test results for Condition X. Using the calculation for PPV (10 true positives/30 total positives), the PPV for this screen is 33% even though the sensitivity and specificity is high. When the prevalence in the general population of Condition X increases to 1 in 100, the PPV increases to 83% (adapted from ACOG, 2016).

Personal Utility

Personal utility is the usefulness of a test for the patient and is completely independent of a test's clinical utility. It is not a measurement that a laboratory can calculate and not something that a genetic counselor can determine. It is the patient's personal view of how a test may be beneficial to her or not and that takes into account her individual goals, morals, and values (Bunnik, 2015; Foster et al., 2009; Grosse, 2010). Personal utility does not have to mean that a diagnosis will be made or ruled out. Personal utility can encompass any reason that a patient may use to decide if they want to pursue a test and can include things like providing reassurance, reducing anxiety, family planning, personal preparation, and future decision-making (Grosse, 2010). A test with very little clinical utility may still have some personal utility and vice versa (Bunnik, 2015; Foster et al., 2009). It is often the role of the genetic counselor to help a patient determine the personal utility—or lack thereof— of a particular test option and to balance that with clinical utility.

Prenatal Screening Options

Fetal prenatal screening is typically divided into two types: maternal serum screening and cell-free DNA (cfDNA) screening (carrier screening will be discussed in Chapter 6).

Maternal Serum Screening

Maternal serum screening, also called *biochemical screening*, is a type of blood test performed on a pregnant woman that estimates the chance that her fetus has Down syndrome, trisomy 18, or an open neural tube defect (ONTD). A detailed explanation of these conditions will not be provided in this text however, refer to Chapter 5 for a summary. Maternal serum screening uses specific analytes found in the mother's blood to provide a probability that the fetus has one of these conditions. Biochemical screening analytes include two maternal serum markers measured in the first trimester: pregnancy-associated plasma protein-A (PAPP-A) and free-beta human chorionic gonadotropin (βhCG); and four measured in the second trimester: alpha-fetoprotein (AFP), total hCG, unconjugated estriol (uE3), and inhibin-A. Maternal serum screening can also include a first-trimester ultrasound measurement called a *nuchal translucency* (NT).

The levels of the analytes measured in the maternal serum change throughout a pregnancy. PAPP-A is a large protein produced by the placenta, and it increases steadily with increasing gestational age (Shiefa, 2012). βhCG is a hormone also produced by the placenta that increases rapidly, peaking at 8–10 weeks and then declining until 18–20 weeks, when it remains steady until the end of pregnancy (Sheifa, 2013). AFP is made by the fetal liver and the yolk sac. It steadily increases throughout pregnancy until about 32 weeks, then rapidly declines. hCG is a hormone produced by the syncytiotrophoblast of the placenta. It increases rapidly during the first 8–10 weeks of gestation, and then it decreases steadily until around 20 weeks, when it remains steady until the end of pregnancy. uE3 is an estrogen hormone produced by the fetal adrenal glands and liver that increases steadily throughout pregnancy (Saller, 1996). Inhibin-A is made mainly by the placenta and increases steadily throughout pregnancy.

NT is a measurement of the fluid-filled space between the fetal spine and the skin of the fetal neck (Driscoll, 2008). The NT increases in size with gestational age. However, it must be measured between 10w0d and 13w6d of gestation as the space loses translucency after 14 weeks and becomes opaque. An NT measurement must be performed by a specially trained sonographer.

Multiples of the Median (MoM)

In prenatal biochemical screening, the actual concentration value of the analytes measured is not what is used to calculate risk. Instead, the values are converted into what is call a *multiple of the median* (MoM). A MoM is calculated by dividing the actual concentration value of a marker, analyte, or NT measurement obtained for a particular patient by the median value of that marker in the population at that gestational age. This is to allow for the natural variation in the concentration of these analytes across pregnancies and for a meaningful comparison of those analytes based on the gestational age of the fetus (Sheifa, 2013). This also allows measurements evaluated by different laboratories to be interpreted consistently. When a person has a marker measurement that is the same as the median level for that marker, the value is 1.0 MoM. All MoMs are compared to a value of 1.0.

Calculating the Risk

An individual risk for aneuploidy is calculated by taking what is called an *a priori risk*, the risk of aneuploidy or ONTD based on what is already known, such as the patient's age and gestational age of the fetus, and adjusting that risk based on the serum analytes and the ultrasound measurements (a likelihood ratio) to provide a new risk estimate.

Risk can be calculated based on a mathematical model. There are many mathematical models used to evaluate risk (of which the specifics will not be discussed), and each laboratory chooses which model it uses. Each model uses the same factors for analysis including maternal age, fetal gestational age (calculated by the crown rump length [CRL]), the concentration values of the analytes, and the ultrasound markers. Other factors are also taken into consideration in the models such as ethnicity, weight, diabetes status, smoking status, the number of fetuses, whether an egg donor was used and the age of the donor, whether the patient had any previous pregnancies with a chromosome abnormality or ONTD, and whether the patient was taking certain types of medication because these can all impact the risk assessment for the conditions being screened. Those with African ancestry, diabetes, a family member with a ONTD, and taking certain medications will increase the *a priori* risk for ONTDs. Maternal age and a previous child with a chromosome abnormality will increase the *a priori* risk for aneuploidy. Inaccurate information provided to the laboratory can lead to inaccurate risk assessment. Each laboratory may also use a different cutoff for a MoM to determine high risk versus low risk for a specific condition. For example, one laboratory may call any result with a greater than 1 in 270 risk for Down syndrome high risk while another laboratory will not call a result high risk until it is greater than 1 in 150. Remember that cutoffs determine the PPV.

Timing and Test Options

Risk assessment is performed on various combinations of first- and second-trimester analyte and ultrasound measurements. There are several ways in which a maternal serum screen can be completed. There are options to complete maternal serum screening only in the first trimester, only in the second trimester, or in a combination of first and second trimesters (Driscoll, 2008). Each option has a unique sensitivity and specificity as well as other benefits and limitations. Determining which version of a test is given to a patient usually depends on the clinic or facility where she is receiving her OB care. Some clinics allow a patient to choose which test she prefers out of all the options, while other clinics may determine the screening method they will use; then the option for the patient is whether to pursue the test or not. Regardless, it is not recommended that patients complete multiple types of maternal serum screening or repeat testing; rather, they should complete a single test to provide a risk assessment.

First-trimester-only screening consists of analysis of PAPP-A and βhCG from maternal serum and ultrasound measurement of NT. For valid analysis, the maternal blood must be drawn and the NT measured between 11w0d and 13w6d (a CRL of 4.4–8.5 cm) (Wald, 1997). Of note, markers analyzed during the first trimester do not screen for open neural tube defects.

Second-trimester-only screening, typically called a *quad screen* or *quadruple screen*, usually consists of analysis of four maternal serum analytes: AFP, hCG, uE3, and inhibin-A (Wald, 1994). Other forms of second-trimester screening exist including a *triple screen* (measurement of AFP, hCG, uE3) and a *penta screen* (measurement of AFP, hCG, uE3, inhibin-A, and ITA [hyperglycosylated hCG]). A Quad/Triple/Penta screen does not include any ultrasound measurements. AFP can also be measured on its own during the second trimester to screen only for open neural tube defects. For valid analysis, the maternal blood must be drawn between 14w0d and 24w6d.

Combined first- and second-trimester screening takes place in the form of an *integrated* or *sequential screen*. Combined screening uses first-trimester maternal serum analytes, PAPP-A, and βhCG, and a NT measurement in addition to second-trimester maternal serum analytes, AFP, hCG, uE3, and inhibin-A to provide a risk assessment. The first part of the test must be completed between 11w0d and 13w6d (a CRL of 4.4–8.5 cm) and the second part between 14w0d and 24w6d. Combined screening has a higher detection rate and a lower false-positive rate (Breathnach et al., 2007; Driscoll, 2008; Metcalfe et al., 2014).

Results

The results for a maternal serum screen are provided as a numeric risk value for each of the two or three conditions being screened. It is usually displayed by stating the individual's *a priori* risk followed by her adjusted risk based on the parameters provided (age, gestational age, etc.) and the cutoff used. Results also typically include the raw concentration value of the marker, MoM values of the marker, the date the blood was drawn, and the parameters provided to the laboratory. See the sample quad screen result in Table 3.2.

Based on the sample result, this individual has an increased risk for her fetus to have Down syndrome. This does not mean that

TABLE 3.2 Example of maternal serum screen results report

	Pre-test risk	Post-test risk	Cutoff
Open neural tube defect	1 in 900	<1 in 10,000	
Down syndrome	1 in 1,100	1 in 35	(1 in 190)
Trisomy 18	1 in 4,600	1 in 2,200	(1 in 100)

INTERPRETATION
Screen positive for Down syndrome

her fetus actually has Down syndrome. In fact, the interpretation of these results suggests that she has a 1 in 35 (2.9%) chance that her fetus has Down syndrome and a 34 in 35 (97.1%) chance that her fetus does *not* have Down syndrome.

Pattern Association

Once the values and the MoMs are established for these markers, how do they translate into an increased or a decreased risk for a chromosome condition? When MoMs are obtained from the markers, the laboratory analyzes those values as a group and not just each value individually. In general, the combination of those MoMs is interpreted based on their overall pattern. Certain patterns of analyte MoMs are associated with an increased risk for a certain condition. See Table 3.3 and Table 3.4 for pattern associations.

TABLE 3.3 Patterns of First-trimester markers

	NT	PAPP-A	βhCG
Down syndrome	High	Low	High
Trisomy 18	High	Low	Low

βhCG, beta human chorionic gonadotropin; NT, nuchal translucency; PAPP-A, pregnancy-associated plasma protein-A.

TABLE 3.4 Patterns of Second-trimester markers

	AFP	hCG	uE3	Inhibin-A
Down syndrome	Low	High	Low	High
Trisomy 18	Low	Low	Low	Low
Open neural tube defect	High	–	–	–

AFP, alpha-fetoprotein; hCG, human chorionic gonadotropin; uE3, unconjugated estriol.

TABLE 3.5 Patterns associated with other fetal conditions

Fetal Conditions	First Trimester			Second Trimester			
	NT	PAPP-A	βhCG	AFP	hCG	uE3	Inhibin-A
Smith-Lemli-Opitz syndrome, X-linked ichthyosis, Congenital adrenal hyperplasia, Placental aromatase deficiency	–	–	–	–	–	Very Low/undetectable	–
Abdominal wall defect	–	–	–	High	–	–	–
Twins	–	High	High	High	High	High	High
Triploidy	–	–	–	–	–	–	Very High
HELLP syndrome	–	–	–	–	–	–	
Loss of one twin	–	–	–	–	–	–	Low
Primary antiphospholipid antibody syndrome	–	–	–	–	–	–	–

AFP, alpha-fetoprotein; βhCG, beta human chorionic gonadotropin; hCG, human chorionic gonadotropin; NT, nuchal translucency; PAPP-A, pregnancy-associated plasma protein-A; uE3, unconjugated estriol.

TABLE 3.6 Patterns associated with adverse pregnancy outcomes

Adverse Pregnancy Outcomes	First trimester			Second trimester			
	NT	PAPP-A	βhCG	AFP	hCG	uE3	Inhibin-A
Intrauterine growth restriction (IUGR)	—	—	—	High	—	—	High
Gestational hypertension (with abnormal maternal uterine Doppler)	—	—	—	—	High	—	—
Preterm birth	—	—	—	—	—	—	—
Miscarriage	—	—	—	—	—	—	—
Spontaneous miscarriage	—	—	Very Low	—	—	—	—
Confined placental mosaic trisomy 16	—	—	—	High	High	—	—
Placental anomaly (molar pregnancy), fetal demise	—	—	Low	—	High	—	—
Preterm birth, stillbirth, miscarriage	—	—	—	Low	—	—	—
Nonspecific adverse obstetrical outcomes (i.e., abruption, preterm birth, stillbirth, low birth weight, membrane rupture)	—	Low	—	Low or High	High	High	Low

AFP, alpha-fetoprotein; βhCG, beta human chorionic gonadotropin; hCG, human chorionic gonadotropin; NT, nuchal translucency; PAPP-A, pregnancy-associated plasma protein-A; uE3, unconjugated estriol.

Although maternal serum analytes and NT measurements are used to screen for Down syndrome, trisomy 18, and neural tube defects, other pattern associations have been noted, such as for other genetic conditions and adverse pregnancy outcomes (i.e., hypertensive disorders during pregnancy, preterm birth, intrauterine growth restriction, perinatal mortality, and placental issues). However, these associations have low sensitivity and high false-positive rates, thus it is not recommended that maternal serum screening be used to identify adverse pregnancy outcomes (Baer et al., 2014, 2015; Craig, 2006; Dugoff et al., 2005; Duric et al., 2003; Gagnon et al., 2008; Huang et al., 2010; Rink, Norton, 2016). See Tables 3.5 and 3.6 for patterns associated with other fetal conditions and adverse outcomes.

An increase in the NT measurement is typically any measurement greater than 3.0 mm, although some centers use a measurement of 2.5 mm (Jackson, Rose, 1998). As discussed earlier, an increase in the NT measurement is a first-trimester marker of aneuploidy, such as Down syndrome, Turner syndrome, and trisomy 18. However, an increased NT measurement may be associated with other chromosome abnormalities, skeletal dysplasias, structural abnormalities such as fetal cardiovascular and pulmonary defects, congenital infection, and metabolic and hematologic disorders (Nicolaides, 2004; Shakoor et al., 2016). In general, the risk for an adverse outcome increases with the size of the NT (Nicolaides, 2004; Scholl et al., 2012) (refer to Chapter 5).

When an increased NT measurement is greater than 5 mm and often septated, it is called a *cystic hygroma*. A cystic hygroma is typically associated with the same types of conditions as an increased NT but since it is a larger measurement, the prognosis is typically poor (even without aneuploidy) (Gedikbasi et al., 2007; Graesslin et al., 2007; Malone, 2005; Scholl et al., 2012; Woodward, 2016). The risk for aneuploidy in a fetus with a cystic hygroma is between 55% and 70% (Woodward, 2016). A cystic hygroma can be detected in either the first or second trimester. When it is seen in the first trimester, the most common aneuploidy is Down syndrome; however, when detected in the second trimester, it is most commonly associated with Turner syndrome (Gedikbasi et al., 2007; Woodward, 2016). In addition to aneuploidy, a single-gene condition called Noonan syndrome is often at the top of the list of differential diagnoses (Alamillo et al., 2012; Graesslin et al., 2007).

Follow-Up of Abnormal Results

When a patient receives an abnormal maternal serum screening test result, she should be offered counseling to discuss the meaning of the result, either by her obstetrician or a genetic counselor, and additional testing options (Jackson, Rose, 1998). The indicated risk will determine which type of testing options are most appropriate. These tests are named here, but further explanation of the tests will be provided in subsequent chapters. Given the gestational age limitations of many of the screens, it is important to confirm that the blood was drawn at the appropriate time and that the correct EDD was used because this can confer a false increased risk result (refer to Chapter 1 for detailed information about gestational age determination).

When a maternal serum screen indicates an increased risk for aneuploidy, the patient should be offered further screening with cfDNA testing or a diagnostic test. An additional ultrasound may also be offered to screen for common defects and markers associated with the aneuploidy (refer to Chapter 5). When a screen indicates an increased risk for an ONTD, an ultrasound should be offered to evaluate for ONTD as well as for other defects, such as in the abdominal wall. The patient should be offered an amniocentesis for evaluation of the fetal AFP level followed by acetylcholinesterase if abnormal (ACOG Practice Bulletin, 2003).

If an increased NT or a cystic hygroma is identified on ultrasound, the patient should be offered genetic counseling and diagnostic testing for aneuploidy as well as a follow-up ultrasound for fetal structural abnormalities (ACOG, 2016). Patients with an enlarged NT or cystic hygroma and normal diagnostic testing for aneuploidy should be offered an anatomic ultrasound evaluation in the second trimester, fetal echocardiography, and further counseling regarding the potential for genetic syndromes not detected by the tests completed (ACOG, 2016).

Of note, it is not recommended for women to be offered further aneuploidy screening after a normal maternal serum screen as it could increase the risk of a false positive (ACOG, 2016).

Limitations of Maternal Serum Screening

As with any testing, there are limitations to maternal serum screening. Proper counseling regarding the benefits and limitations of each testing option should be provided to the patient in order for her to make an informed choice (Chard, Norton, 2016). First and most importantly, a screen is designed only to evaluate the risk for a condition; it cannot diagnose a fetus with a specific condition. The screen is only designed to screen for certain conditions, as discussed earlier, and is not validated to provide information on other conditions. This means that maternal serum screening cannot provide risk estimates for other aneuploidies such as trisomy 13, Turner syndrome, other sex chromosome aneuploidies, or triploidy. These tests cannot provide information on microdeletion or microduplication syndromes or most single-gene disorders.

There are technical and biological limitations of maternal serum screening. Many complexities arise with twin pregnancies including determination of zygosity in same-sex dichorionic gestations. In dizygotic twins, the risk for each fetus is independent; however, with some rare exceptions, in monozygotic twins, the risk is the same for each fetus. This means that one twin in a di-di gestation may have an aneuploidy when the other does not, whereas in mono-mono gestations both fetuses are typically either affected or not. Serum markers are approximately twice as high in twin pregnancies as in singletons but not exactly double (Rink, Norton, 2016). Since maternal serum screening relies on analytes found in maternal blood, there is no way to determine how much of each analyte is being contributed by each fetus. The exception is a NT measurement, which is independent and specific for each fetus regardless of zygosity (Audibert, 2011; Prats, 2012; Rink, Norton, 2016; Wald et al., 2003). Thus, a twin with a normal chromosome complement can mask aneuploidy in the other twin (Muller et al., 2003). This results in lower detection rates for maternal serum screening in twin pregnancies than in singleton pregnancies (Audibert, 2011; Wald et al., 2003). Maternal serum screening is not recommended in women with higher order multiple gestations given the limited data on performance. Maternal serum screening should be discouraged when a woman experiences a loss of one twin early in gestation while the other twin survives (ACOG, 2016). This is because the death of the twin may be related to a genetic condition or aneuploidy as well as the fact that a demise increases some serum analytes, which could result in a falsely increased risk result for the live twin.

Obesity can affect many aspects of a woman's pregnancy including prenatal screening. Obesity is defined as a body mass index (BMI) of 30 or greater (Rose, 2016). In general, the levels of PAPP-A, βhCG, Ue3, AFP, inhibin, and hCG decrease as a woman's weight increases (Palomaki et al., 1990; Spencer et al., 2003). This decrease is assumed to be due to the dilutional effect of those analytes in a larger blood volume in the patient. Therefore, weight is one of the factors that can impact the test's risk estimate and is provided to the laboratory for use in their algorithm. Laboratories typically have a maximum weight that their algorithm can incorporate (Rose, 2015). When a patient weighs more than this, the results of the screen become less accurate. In addition to the effect that weight has on the analytes measured in the maternal blood, NT measurement can also be impacted by being overweight. A first-trimester ultrasound in an obese patient is limited in its ability to provide a good view of the fetus, which can result in the inability to obtain an NT measurement or a significant increase in the time needed to obtain it (Rose, 2015).

Vaginal bleeding during the first trimester can occur in many pregnancies without the result of miscarriage. However, first-trimester bleeding has been shown to have an impact on the results of maternal serum screening. It has been noted that βhCG levels in the first trimester and AFP levels in the second trimester increase when a woman had an episode of first-trimester bleeding (Berry, 1995; De Biasio et al., 2003). This increase can impact the risk assessment provided by maternal serum screening results.

Cell-Free DNA Testing

cfDNA screening goes by many names. It is also commonly known as *noninvasive prenatal testing (NIPT)* or *noninvasive prenatal screening (NIPS)*. Historically, it was termed *noninvasive prenatal diagnosis (NIPD)*, which is incorrect as it is not a diagnostic test. Additionally, it is often described by its brand name, which varies depending on what company offers the test. Given that NIPT and NIPS are nonspecific terms and that brand names are company-specific, we prefer to use cfDNA to describe this form of screening.

Origin

Both cell-free fetal and cell-free maternal DNA circulate in maternal plasma (Lo et al., 1997). See Figure 3.2. The maternal and fetal cfDNA are free from a cell, circulate as short fragments

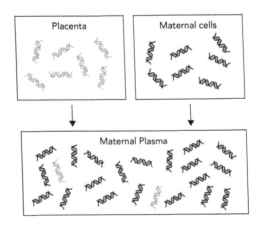

FIGURE 3.2

Origin of cell-free DNA.

(<200 base pairs), and are representative of the entire genome (Chan et al., 2004). The maternal cfDNA originates primarily from apoptosis of maternal hematopoietic cells (precursor blood cells) and adipocytes (fat cells) (Lui et al., 2002). The primary source of fetal cfDNA is thought to be from apoptosis of placental cells.

The significance of the origin of the fetal cfDNA is that the placenta and the fetus do not always correspond genetically. Although the egg and sperm join to create the fetus and extraembryonic tissues (including the placenta), mosaicism may arise including either true fetal mosaicism or confined placental mosaicism. These situations have been known to lead to discrepancies between test results and fetal status (Canick et al., 2013; Grati, 2016) and are therefore a source of false negatives and false positives.

Another source of incorrect or uninterpretable test results is the presence of maternal conditions. Given that maternal DNA is also in the sample, testing has the potential to identify maternal sex chromosome abnormalities (e.g., 47,XXX), maternal microdeletion (22q11.2 deletion syndrome), maternal somatic cell variation (natural loss of an X chromosome with maternal age), and maternal malignancy (Osborne et al., 2013; Wang et al., 2015; Wang et al., 2014). The patient should be informed of this limitation. Current guidelines offer little assistance in the event of uninterpretable results, but further clinical evaluation may be considered including maternal karyotype if warranted (see Chapter 4 for discussion of karyotyping).

Fetal Fraction

The contribution of cfDNA in a maternal blood sample that is fetal in origin is termed the *fetal fraction*. Although there is substantial sample-to-sample variation, fetal DNA comprises approximately 3–13% of the total circulating cfDNA in maternal plasma

(Lo et al., 1998). The fetal fraction increases with advancing gestational age, averaging 0.1% per week up to 20 weeks' gestation. After 20 weeks, it increases at about 1% per week until delivery (Wang et al., 2013).

Having enough fetal cfDNA available in a sample is crucial for test performance and understanding results. Many factors can reduce the amount observed, including early gestational age, increased maternal weight or BMI (Ashoor et al., 2013; Vora et al., 2012; Wang et al., 2013), and fetal aneuploidy (Norton, Wapner, 2015; Pergament et al., 2014). In patients with significant obesity, other forms of screening should be offered and the limitations of cfDNA testing should be discussed (Gregg et al., 2016). Given the concern for an increased risk of chromosome abnormalities with a low fetal fraction, the ACOG and the Society for Maternal Fetal Medicine (SMFM) (Committee Opinion No 640) as well as the American College of Medical Genetics and Genomics (ACMG) (Gregg et al., 2016) recommend that any patient receiving a "no-call" result from cfDNA testing should be offered further genetic counseling and be offered a comprehensive ultrasound and diagnostic testing. Although repeat cfDNA testing could also be considered, this may delay a diagnosis, which in turn may limit the patient's reproductive options. Therefore, repeat cfDNA testing is currently not recommended by ACMG.

Clearance

Fetal cfDNA is cleared from maternal plasma in a relatively short amount of time after delivery. The half-life has been reported at 1 hour. There is almost complete clearance occurring between 1 and 2 days postpartum (Lo et al., 1999; Yu et al., 2013). Given that the cfDNA present in maternal circulation from a pregnancy will be cleared before the patient has any subsequent pregnancies, any previous pregnancy is not expected to alter the results of a current one.

Methodology

In general, currently there are two methods for analyzing cfDNA, a quantitative "counting" method or a single nucleotide polymorphism (SNP)-based method. Although the techniques vary, both involve analyzing the mixture of fetal and maternal cfDNA in the maternal blood sample and amplifying the cfDNA, followed by the use of next-generation sequencing (NGS) technology and application of advanced bioinformatic analyses for interpretation.

The counting method can be further broken down to two approaches: *massively parallel shotgun sequencing (MPSS)* or *targeted sequencing*. MPSS allows for sequencing large numbers (tens of millions) of small DNA sequences, or fragments, from the entire genome. These are random fragments representative of all the chromosomes that are sequenced simultaneously in a single run, and therefore not all reads will be useful in the analysis. Alternatively, sequencing can be done using a targeted approach. Targeted sequencing selectively amplifies the genomic regions of interest, thus creating a more efficient process in which all the reads are used in the test interpretation (please see Figure 3.3).

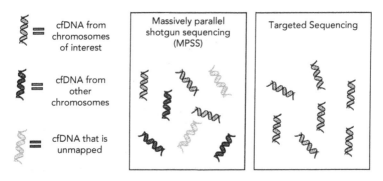

FIGURE 3.3

Massively parallel shotgun sequencing (MPSS) versus targeted sequencing.

The next step after amplification and sequencing is to determine the chromosome origin of each DNA fragment. Since the sequence of the whole genome is known, this can be done by comparing the sequence data from each fragment to a human genome reference. Afterward, the amount of fragments that map to any given chromosome can be quantified and compared to the number of fragments that map to a reference chromosome from the sample, which is presumably euploid. If the fetus is euploid, the ratio of fragments from the chromosome of interest compared to the fragments from the reference chromosome will be as expected. If the fetus is trisomic, then there will be more genetic material originating from the extra chromosome, thus altering the ratio observed (Chiu, et al. 2008). Please see Figure 3.4.

In contrast, the SNP-based method determines copy number by observing specific patterns in allelic measurements. First, targeted sequencing of thousands of SNPs on chromosomes of interest is completed. SNPs are normal genetic variations within a population. They are differences in single nucleotides at particular positions throughout the genome. For example, perhaps within a population most people have the base A at a particular position, but some have the base C at this position. People with the A would be said to have allele A. People with the less common base C would be said to have allele B. Since we have two alleles for any particular locus, a person's allele pattern would be able to be determined as AA, AB, or BB. Fetuses that are trisomic could be AAA, AAB, ABB, or BBB at that locus. Each locus is analyzed for the allelic measurements and then an advanced system, called the *next-generation aneuploidy test using SNPs (NATUS)* algorithm, considers parental genotypes and HapMap crossover frequency data to determine millions of hypotheses for possible fetal chromosome number. The fetal–maternal DNA pattern is then compared to each of these hypotheses to find the closest match using a Bayesian-based maximum likelihood statistical method (Nicolaides et al., 2013). Please see Figure 3.5.

The SNP-based method has the advantage of being able to detect triploidy and vanishing twins (but currently cannot

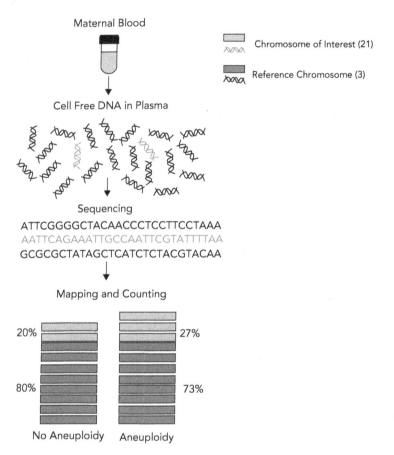

FIGURE 3.4

Counting method.

determine the difference between the two) as well as effectively differentiate between maternal and fetal cfDNA, which is important in situations in which maternal conditions are present. However, this method is limited in that it currently cannot be used in cases of multiples and for women who are not the biological mothers of the fetus (if the mother used a donor egg or if a surrogate is used).

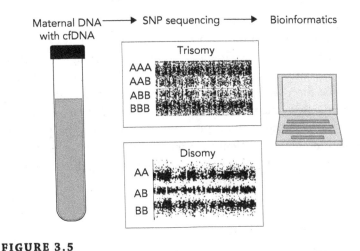

FIGURE 3.5

Single nucleotide polymorphism (SNP) method.

Conditions Analyzed

Common chromosome abnormalities including Down syndrome (T21), trisomy 18 (T18), and trisomy 13 (T13) are most commonly evaluated with the use of cfDNA. Many patients also value the ability of the test to predict fetal sex. This is clinically useful when a patient is a known carrier of an X-linked condition and fetal gender may alter their decision to pursue diagnostic testing. Many laboratories also offer analysis of sex chromosome abnormalities including monosomy X (45,X), Klinefelter syndrome (47,XXY), triple X syndrome (47,XXX), and Jacobs syndrome (47,XYY). Some laboratories offer evaluation of fetal Rh status when alloimmunization is of concern, evaluation of triploidy or a vanishing twin, a select set of microdeletion syndromes (e.g., Prader Willi, Angelman, Cri-Du-Chat, 22q11.2 deletions, 1p36 deletion, Wolf-Hirschhorn, Langer-Giedion, and Jacobsen), other autosomal aneuploidies (e.g., trisomy 22, trisomy 16), and even evaluation of genome-wide copy number variation of 7 megabases or more. Although clinically available, current guidelines do not recommend testing for microdeletions, other autosomal trisomies, or genome-wide testing (Committee Opinion no. 640, 2015; Committee Opinion no. 682, 2016; Gregg et al., 2016). Although a clinician may make this available to patients, the limitations of testing should be discussed. Additionally, although research has shown that clinically available cfDNA testing can be used to detect some monogenic conditions and is now currently available for providers to offer and order for patients (Amicucci et al., 2000; Guissart et al., 2016; Parks et al., 2016), at the time of this writing, this testing not yet recommended by guidelines.

Test Performance

Although laboratories vary, all tests have relatively high sensitivities and specificities for T21 and T18 regardless of the method used. The accuracy of testing for T13 is generally lower. A recent meta-analysis (Iwarsson et al., 2017) combined information from multiple studies for evaluation of both the general pregnant population as well as those with high-risk pregnancies. This review reported, for the high-risk population, a pooled sensitivity for T21 of 99.8%, T18 of 97.7%, and T13 of 97.5%. In the average-risk population, the pooled sensitivity for T21 was 99.3%. Due to the low number of studies for the average-risk population, the sensitivity and specificity for T18 and T13 could not be calculated. However, other studies have indicated similar sensitivities and specificities of trisomy 21 and 18 in the general obstetric population (Bianchi et al., 2014; Nicolaides et al., 2012).

The sex chromosome abnormalities have also been studied. In 2015, a meta-analysis (Gil et al., 2015) mostly consisting of people in the high-risk population, which included a total of 16 studies, for a combined total of 177 singleton pregnancies with fetal monosomy X and 9,079 without monosomy X to give a pooled detection rate of 90.2% and a false-positive rate of 0.23%. For sex chromosome abnormalities other than monosomy X, 12 studies with 56 affected and 6,699 non–sex chromosome abnormality pregnancies were used for a pooled detection rate of 93% and a false-positive rate of 0.14%. Given this, it appears that the detection rate is greater than 90% and the false-positive rate is less than 1%.

Who To Offer Testing To?

Testing by cfDNA first became clinically available in 2011. In 2012 (Committee Opinion no. 545, 2012), the ACOG and SMFM recommended offering testing only to women with an increased risk of aneuploidy. This included women who are 35 years or older at the time of delivery, patients with a history of a prior affected pregnancy or child, patients whose current pregnancy was identified with ultrasound findings consistent with an increased risk of aneuploidy, when either parent was a carrier of a balanced Robertsonian translocation involving chromosomes 21 or 13, and those with abnormal maternal serum screening. In 2016, an updated statement from ACOG and SMFM was issued (Committee Opinion no. 640, 2015) suggesting that cfDNA screening should be made available both to patients in the high-risk population and to those in the average-risk population. However, those in the average-risk population should be made aware of the limitations, including the lower PPV and its inability to detect adverse pregnancy outcomes. In 2016, the ACMG (Gregg et al., 2016) published a statement recommending that all pregnant patients be offered cfDNA testing. Given this, at this time, any patient can elect to pursue cfDNA testing, but she should be made aware of its limitations, benefits, risks, and alternatives.

Multiples and Vanishing Twins

Although laboratories offer cfDNA testing for multiples (e.g., twins, triplets), it is currently not recommended (Committee Opinion no. 640, 2015; Gregg et al., 2016; Practice Bulletin no. 163, 2016). This is due to the limited availability of data on test performance. Although more data are needed, published studies have suggested detection rates similar to those of singletons (Gil, 2015; Huang et al., 2014). cfDNA screening by a maternal blood specimen for aneuploidy in multiples is complicated, however, due to the fact it can only provide a single combined result for the entire pregnancy, without the ability to distinguish risk between fetuses. This is particularly important for dizygotic twins, where it can lead to situations of incorrect test result in regards to aneuploidy status or fetal sex (Kelley et al., 2016). Similarly, patients with a vanishing twin or twin demise have higher likelihoods of incorrect test results on cfDNA testing (Grömminger et al., 2014). More false positives would be expected given the high rate of aneuploidy in first-trimester miscarriages (Menasha et al., 2005). In the event of a known twin demise/vanishing twin or when one twin has an anomaly identified by ultrasound, screening should be discouraged and diagnostic testing should be offered.

Adverse Pregnancy Outcomes

Testing by cfDNA cannot be used to detect ONTDs or pregnancy complications. Given this, for any patient electing this testing, it is recommended to offer a maternal serum AFP screen in the second trimester. (Please see the maternal serum screening section for further details on this option.)

Considerations Prior to Testing

Prior to testing, a detailed pregnancy and family history should be obtained to determine if this form of testing is the most appropriate for the patient. Guidelines (Gregg et al., 2016) recommend completing a baseline ultrasound to confirm gestational age and viability and to identify multiples. Clinical considerations such as ultrasound findings and likelihood for conditions being tested should also be considered. For example, cfDNA testing is not an appropriate test for a patient with a reciprocal translocation of chromosomes 11 and 22 or for a patient with a fetus that has findings suggestive of a skeletal dysplasia. In fact, any patient with a structural anomaly identified on ultrasound should be offered diagnostic testing.

Results and Follow-up

After testing, most people will find themselves in one of two categories. Either a patient will have a negative screen and her posttest risk of having a baby with an aneuploidy will be lower than her pretest risk, or she will have a positive screen and will be at an increased risk of having a baby with an aneuploidy. In the event of negative results, the patient should be notified that a residual risk still exists. Additional aneuploidy screening (e.g., the quad screen) should not be offered when a patient has a negative screen because it can lead to more false positives. Patients with normal screenings may still elect to go on to have a diagnostic procedure (amniocentesis or chorionic villus sampling [CVS]). Although the patient can pursue diagnostic testing due to her own preference and desire, this is particularly relevant to patients who completed screening early in their pregnancy but are later identified with additional findings such as ultrasound abnormalities. Normal cfDNA testing does not replace the need for an anatomy scan between 18 and 20 weeks of pregnancy.

Alternatively for those receiving abnormal results, patients will often want to know what the specific likelihood is that their baby has the condition of interest. Although, it is recommended (Committee Opinion no. 640, 2015) that cfDNA testing laboratories report PPVs, many do not provide this information. This is due to the complexity of incorporating multiple factors into the risk analysis, including age, gestational age, and ultrasound findings. PPV can be calculated using a bayesian analysis. Any other questions that arise about the condition of concern or management should also be addressed.

It is recommended that any patient with an abnormal cfDNA test be offered confirmatory diagnostic testing. Please see Chapter 4 for more information about these options. Although it is always the patient's choice whether or not to have a diagnostic test, it is highly recommended should the patient be considering an irreversible action such as pregnancy termination (Committee Opinion no. 640, 2015; Gregg et al., 2016).

Most patients will pursue cfDNA testing in the first trimester before an anatomy ultrasound has been completed. In these situations, ultrasound may be offered to provide additional information prior to pursuing diagnostic testing. The utility of the ultrasound is limited by gestational age. Anatomy scans are most informative at 18–20 weeks, but waiting until this age could delay a diagnosis. Therefore, although an early scan could be considered, structural anomalies may be missed. It should be stressed that although an ultrasound may be useful in helping with interpretation of test results, it does not replace the use of diagnostic testing.

Should a patient decline diagnostic testing, further testing after the completion of the pregnancy should be pursued. Given the limitations of cfDNA to differentiate between a trisomy or translocation, a fetal karyotype on either the products of conception or a sample of cord blood should be completed.

Resources

The National Society of Genetic Counselors (NSGC) and the Perinatal Quality Foundation have created a calculator to assist providers in estimating the PPV and NPV of cfDNA screening. This tool has been endorsed by the ACOG and the SMFM. In addition to the calculator, there is a list of resources including information on cfDNA and links to patient support groups and professional organizations. As of publication, these can be at www.perinatalquality.org/Vendors/NSGC/NIPT/.

Conclusion

Understanding the details of the basic screening options during pregnancy, as well as mastering the ability to evaluate the usefulness of a screen, is an integral part of perinatal genetic counseling.

A perinatal counselor must fully understand the differences between testing options, including benefits and limitations, and they must be able to explain these options to a patient who has very little or no previous knowledge or understanding of these concepts. Translation of this complex information into a patient-friendly format is a skill that every perinatal genetic counselor must master. The counselor must assess whether a test is clinically indicated and appropriate as well as help the patient to make a decision about the testing that is best for her.

References

ACOG Practice Bulletin. Neural tube defects. Number 44. *Int J Gynaecol Obstet*. 2003 Oct;83(1):123–133.

Alamillo CM, Fiddler M, Pergament E. Increased nuchal translucency in the presence of normal chromosomes: what's next? *Curr Opin Obstet Gynecol*. 2012 Mar;24(2):102–108.

Amicucci P, Gennarelli M, Novelli G, Dallapiccola B. Prenatal diagnosis of myotonic dystrophy using fetal DNA obtained from maternal plasma. *Clin Chem*. 2000 Feb;46(2):301–302.

Ashoor G, Syngelaki A, Poon LC, Rezende JC, Nicolaides KH. Fetal fraction in maternal plasma cell-free DNA at 11–13 weeks' gestation: relation to maternal and fetal characteristics. *Ultrasound Obstet Gynecol*. 2013 Jan;41(1):26–32.

Audibert F, Gagnon A; Genetics Committee of the Society of Obstetricians and Gynaecologists of Canada; Prenatal Diagnosis Committee of the Canadian College of Medical Geneticists. Prenatal screening for and diagnosis of aneuploidy in twin pregnancies. *J Obstet Gynaecol Can*. 2011 Jul;33(7):754–767.

Baer RJ, Currier RJ, Norton ME, Flessel MC, Goldman S, Towner D, Jelliffe-Pawlowski LL. Obstetric, perinatal, and fetal outcomes in pregnancies with false-positive integrated screening results. *Obstet Gynecol*. 2014 Mar;123(3):603–609.

Baer RJ, Flessel MC, Jelliffe-Pawlowski LL, Goldman S, Hudgins L, Hull AD, Norton ME, Currier RJ. Detection rates for aneuploidy by first-trimester and sequential screening. *Obstet Gynecol*. 2015 Oct;126(4):753–759.

Bianchi DW, Parker RL, Wentworth J, Madankumar R, Saffer C, Das AF, Craig JA, Chudova DI, Devers PL, Jones KW, Oliver K, Rava RP, Sehnert AJ; CARE Study Group. DNA sequencing versus standard prenatal aneuploidy screening. *N Engl J Med.* 2014 Feb 27;370(9):799–808.

Berry E, Aitken DA, Crossley JA, Macri JN, Connor JM. Analysis of maternal serum alpha-fetoprotein and free beta human chorionic gonadotrophin in the first trimester: implications for Down's syndrome screening. *Prenat Diagn.* 1995 Jun;15(6):555–565.

Breathnach FM, Malone FD, Lambert-Messerlian G, Cuckle HS, Porter TF, Nyberg DA, et al. First- and second-trimester screening: detection of aneuploidies other than Down syndrome. *Obstet Gynecol.* 2007 Sep;110(3):651–657.

Bunnik EM, Janssens AC, Schermer MH. Personal utility in genomic testing: is there such a thing? *J Med Ethics.* 2015 Apr;41(4):322–326.

Canick JA, Palomaki GE, Kloza EM, Lambert-Messerlian GM, Haddow JE. The impact of maternal plasma DNA fetal fraction on next generation sequencing tests for common fetal aneuploidies. *Prenat Diagn.* 2013 Jul;33(7):667–674.

Chan KC, Zhang J, Hui AB, Wong N, Lau TK, Leung TN, Lo KW, Huang DW, Lo YM. Size distributions of maternal and fetal DNA in maternal plasma. *Clin Chem.* 2004 Jan;50(1):88–92.

Chard RL, Norton ME. Genetic counseling for patients considering screening and diagnosis for chromosomal abnormalities. *Clin Lab Med.* 2016 Jun;36(2):227–236.

Chiu RW, Chan KC, Gao Y, Lau VY, Zheng W, Leung TY, Foo CH, Xie B, Tsui NB, Lun FM, Zee BC, Lau TK, Cantor CR, Lo YM. Noninvasive prenatal diagnosis of fetal chromosomal aneuploidy by massively parallel genomic sequencing of DNA in maternal plasma. *Proc Natl Acad Sci U S A.* 2008 Dec 23;105(51):20458–20463.

Committee Opinion no. 545: Noninvasive prenatal testing for fetal aneuploidy. *Obstet Gynecol.* 2012 Dec;120(6):1532–1534.

Committee Opinion no. 640: Cell-free DNA screening for fetal aneuploidy. *Obstet Gynecol.* 2015 Sep;126(3):e31–e37.

Committee Opinion no. 682: Microarrays and next-generation sequencing technology: the use of advanced genetic diagnostic tools in obstetrics and gynecology. *Obstet Gynecol.* 2016 Dec;128(6):e262–e268.

Craig WY, Haddow JE, Palomaki GE, Kelley RI, Kratz LE, Shackleton CH, Marcos J, Stephen Tint G, MacRae AR, Nowaczyk MJ, Kloza EM, Irons MB, Roberson M. Identifying Smith-Lemli-Opitz syndrome in conjunction with prenatal screening for Down syndrome. *Prenat Diagn*. 2006 Sep;26(9):842–849.

De Biasio P, Canini S, Crovo A, Prefumo F, Venturini PL. Early vaginal bleeding and first-trimester markers for Down syndrome. *Prenat Diagn*. 2003 Jun;23(6):470–473.

Driscoll DA, Gross SJ; Professional Practice and Guidelines Committee. First trimester diagnosis and screening for fetal aneuploidy. Genet Med. 2008 Jan;10(1):73–75.

Dugoff L, Hobbins JC, Malone FD, Vidaver J, Sullivan L, Canick JA, Lambert-Messerlian GM, Porter TF, Luthy DA, Comstock CH, Saade G, Eddleman K, Merkatz IR, Craigo SD, Timor-Tritsch IE, Carr SR, Wolfe HM, D'Alton ME; FASTER Trial Research Consortium. Quad screen as a predictor of adverse pregnancy outcome. *Obstet Gynecol*. 2005 Aug;106(2):260–267.

Duric K, Skrablin S, Lesin J, Kalafatic D, Kuvacic I, Suchanek E. Second trimester total human chorionic gonadotropin, alpha-fetoprotein and unconjugated estriol in predicting pregnancy complications other than fetal aneuploidy. *Eur J Obstet Gynecol Reprod Biol*. 2003 Sep 10;110(1):12–15.

Foster MW, Mulvihill JJ, Sharp RR. Evaluating the utility of personal genomic information. *Genet Med*. 2009 Aug;11(8):570–574.

Gagnon A, Wilson RD, Audibert F, Allen VM, Blight C, Brock JA, Désilets VA, Johnson JA, Langlois S, Summers A, Wyatt P; Society of Obstetricians and Gynaecologists of Canada Genetics Committee. Obstetrical complications associated with abnormal maternal serum markers analytes. *J Obstet Gynaecol Can*. 2008 Oct;30(10):918–949.

Gil MM, Quezada MS, Revello R, Akolekar R, Nicolaides KH. Analysis of cell-free DNA in maternal blood in screening for fetal aneuploidies: updated meta-analysis. *Ultrasound Obstet Gynecol*. 2015 Mar;45(3):249–266. doi:10.1002/uog.14791. Epub 2015 Feb 1.

Gedikbasi A, Gul A, Sargin A, Ceylan Y. Cystic hygroma and lymphangioma: associated findings, perinatal outcome and prognostic factors in live-born infants. *Arch Gynecol Obstet*. 2007 Nov;276(5):491–498.

Graesslin O, Derniaux E, Alanio E, Gaillard D, Vitry F, Quéreux C, Ducarme G. Characteristics and outcome of fetal cystic hygroma diagnosed in the first trimester. *Acta Obstet Gynecol Scand.* 2007;86(12):1442–1446.

Grati FR. Implications of fetoplacental mosaicism on cell-free DNA testing: a review of a common biological phenomenon. *Ultrasound Obstet Gynecol.* 2016 Oct;48(4):415–423.

Gregg AR, Skotko BG, Benkendorf JL, Monaghan KG, Bajaj K, Best RG, Klugman S, Watson MS. Noninvasive prenatal screening for fetal aneuploidy, 2016 update: a position statement of the American College of Medical Genetics and Genomics. *Genet Med.* 2016 Oct;18(10):1056–1065.

Grömminger S, Yagmur E, Erkan S, Nagy S, Schöck U, Bonnet J, Smerdka P, Ehrich M, Wegner RD, Hofmann W, Stumm M. Fetal aneuploidy detection by cell-free DNA sequencing for multiple pregnancies and quality issues with vanishing twins. *J Clin Med.* 2014 Jun 25;3(3):679–692.

Grosse SD, Kalman L, Khoury MJ. Evaluation of the validity and utility of genetic testing for rare diseases. *Ady Exp Med Biol.* 2010;686:115–131.

Guissart C, Dubucs C, Raynal C, Girardet A, Tran Mau Them F, Debant V, Rouzier C, Boureau-Wirth A, Haquet E, Puechberty J, Bieth E, Dupin Deguine D, Khau Van Kien P, Brechard MP, Pritchard V, Koenig M, Claustres M, Vincent MC. Non-invasive prenatal diagnosis (NIPD) of cystic fibrosis: an optimized protocol using MEMO fluorescent PCR to detect the p.Phe508del mutation. *J Cyst Fibros.* 2016 Dec 28. Pii: S1569–1993(16)30680–30684. https://www.perinatalquality.org/Vendors/NSGC/NIPT/

Guttmacher AE, Collins FS, Carmona RH. The Family History-more important than ever. *N Engl J Med.* 2004 Nov 25;351(22):2333–2336.

Huang T, Hoffman B, Meschino W, Kingdom J, Okun N. Prediction of adverse pregnancy outcomes by combinations of first and second trimester biochemistry markers used in the routine prenatal screening of Down syndrome. *Prenat Diagn.* 2010 May;30(5):471–477.

Huang X, Zheng J, Chen M, Zhao Y, Zhang C, Liu L, Xie W, Shi S, Wei Y, Lei D, Xu C, Wu Q, Guo X, Shi X, Zhou Y, Liu Q, Gao Y, Jiang F, Zhang H, Su F, Ge H, Li X, Pan X, Chen S, Chen F, Fang Q, Jiang H, Lau TK, Wang W. Noninvasive prenatal testing of trisomies 21 and 18 by massively parallel sequencing of maternal plasma DNA in twin pregnancies. *Prenat Diagn.* 2014 Apr;34(4):335–340.

Iwarsson E, Jacobsson B, Dagerhamn J, Davidson T, Bernabé E, Heibert Arnlind M. Analysis of cell-free fetal DNA in maternal blood for detection of trisomy 21, 18 and 13 in a general pregnant population and in a high risk population—a systematic review and meta-analysis. *Acta Obstet Gynecol Scand.* 2017 Jan;96(1):7–18.

Jackson M, Rose NC. Diagnosis and management of fetal nuchal translucency. *Semin Roentgenol.* 1998 Oct;33(4):333–338.

Kelley JF, Henning G, Ambrose A, Adelman A. Vanished Twins and Misdiagnosed Sex: A Case Report with Implications in Prenatal Counseling Using Noninvasive Cell-Free DNA Screening. *J Am Board Fam Med.* 2016 May–Jun;29(3):411–413.

Lalkhen A, McClusky A. Clinical tests: sensitivity and specificity. *Contin Educ Anaesth Crit Care Pain.* 2008;8(6):221–223.

Lo YM, Corbetta N, Chamberlain PF. Presence of fetal DNA in maternal plasma and serum. *Lancet.* 1997;350:485.

Lo YM, Zhang J, Leung TN, Lau TK, Chang AM, Hjelm NM. Rapid clearance of fetal DNA from maternal plasma. *Am J Hum Genet.* 1999;64:218–224.

Loong TW. Understanding sensitivity and specificity with the right side of the brain. *BMJ.* 2003 Sep 27;327(7417):716–719.

Lui YY, Chik KW, Chiu RW. Predominant hematopoietic origin of cell-free DNA in plasma and serum after sex-mismatched bone marrow transplantation. *Clin Chem.* 2002;48:421. Mar;24(2):102–8.

Malone FD, Ball RH, Nyberg DA, Comstock CH, Saade GR, Berkowitz RL,et al. First-trimester septated cystic hygroma: prevalence, natural history, and pediatric outcome. *Obstet Gynecol.* 2005 Aug;106(2):288–294.

Menasha J, Levy B, Hirschhorn K, Kardon NB. Incidence and spectrum of chromosome abnormalities in spontaneous abortions: new insights from a 12-year study. *Genet Med.* 2005;7:251–263.

Metcalfe A, Hippman C, Pastuck M, Johnson JA. Beyond trisomy 21: additional chromosomal anomalies detected through routine aneuploidy screening. *J Clin Med.* 2014 Apr 8;3(2):388–415.

Muller F, Dreux S, Dupoizat H. Second trimester Down syndrome maternal serum screening in twin pregnancies: impact of chorionicity. *Prenat Diagn.* 2003;23:331–335.

Nicolaides KH, Syngelaki A, Ashoor G, Birdir C, Touzet G. Noninvasive prenatal testing for fetal trisomies in a routinely screened first-trimester population. *Am J Obstet Gynecol.* 2012 Nov;207(5):374.e1–e6.

Nicolaides KH, Syngelaki A, Gil M, Atanasova V, Markova D. Validation of targeted sequencing of single-nucleotide polymorphisms for non-invasive prenatal detection of aneuploidy of chromosomes 13, 18, 21, X, and Y. *Prenat Diagn.* 2013 Jun;33(6):575–579.

Nicolaides KH. Nuchal translucency and other first-trimester sonographic markers of chromosomal abnormalities. *Am J Obstet Gynecol.* 2004 Jul;191(1):45–67.

Norton ME, Wapner RJ. Cell-free DNA analysis for noninvasive examination of trisomy. *N Engl J Med.* 2015 Dec 24;373(26):2582.

Osborne CM, Hardisty E, Devers P, Kaiser-Rogers K, Hayden MA, Goodnight W, Vora NL. Discordant noninvasive prenatal testing results in a patient subsequently diagnosed with metastatic disease. *Prenat Diagn.* 2013 Jun;33(6):609–611.

Palomaki GE, Panizza DS, Canick JA. Screening for Down syndrome using AFP, uE3 and hCG: effect of maternal weight. *Am J Hum Genet.* 1990;7:a282.

Parks M, Court S, Cleary S, Clokie S, Hewitt J, Williams D, Cole T, MacDonald F, Griffiths M, Allen S. Non-invasive prenatal diagnosis of Duchenne and Becker muscular dystrophies by relative haplotype dosage. *Prenat Diagn.* 2016 Apr;36(4):312–320.

Pergament E, Cuckle H, Zimmermann B, Banjevic M, Sigurjonsson S, Ryan A. Single-nucleotide polymorphism-based noninvasive prenatal screening in a high-risk and low-risk cohort. *Obstet Gynecol.* 2014;124:210–218.

American College of Gynecology and Obstetrics. Practice Bulletin no. 163 Summary: Screening for fetal aneuploidy. *Obstet Gynecol.* 2016 May;127(5):979–981.

Prats P, Rodríguez I, Comas C, Puerto B. First trimester risk assessment for trisomy 21 in twin pregnancies combining nuchal translucency and first trimester biochemical markers. *Prenat Diagn.* 2012 Oct;32(10):927–932.

Rink BD, Norton ME. Screening for fetal aneuploidy. *Semin Perinatol.* 2016 Feb;40(1):35–43.

Rose NC. Genetic screening and the obese gravida. *Clin Obstet Gynecol.* 2016 Mar;59(1):140–147.

Saller DN, Canick JA. Maternal serum screening for fetal Down syndrome:clinical aspects. *Clin Obstet Gynecol.* 1996 Dec;39(4):783–792.

Scholl J, Durfee SM, Russell MA, Heard AJ, Iyer C, Alammari R, Coletta J, Craigo SD, Fuchs KM, D'Alton M, House M, Jennings RW, Ecker J, Panda B, Tanner C, Wolfberg A, Benson CB. First-trimester cystic hygroma: relationship of nuchal translucency thickness and outcomes. *Obstet Gynecol.* 2012 Sep;120(3):551–559.

Shakoor S, Dileep D, Tirmizi S, Rashid S, Amin Y, Munim S. Increased nuchal translucency and adverse pregnancy outcomes. *J Matern Fetal Neonatal Med.* 2016 Sep 5:1–4.

Shiefa S, Amargandhi M, Bhupendra J, Moulali S, Kristine T. First trimester maternal serum screening using biochemical markers PAPP-A and free β-hCG for Down Syndrome, Patau Syndrome and Edward Syndrome. *Indian Journal of Clinical Biochemistry.* 2012 Oct 12;28(1):3–12.

Spencer K, Bindra R, Nicolaides KH. Maternal weight correction of maternal serum PAPP-A and free beta-hCG MoM when screening for trisomy 21 in the first trimester. *Prenat Diagn.* 2003;23:851–855.

Vora NL, Johnson KL, Basu S. A multifactorial relationship exists between total circulating cell-free DNA levels and maternal BMI. *Prenat Diagn* 2012;32:912–914.

Wald NJ, Densem JW, Smith D, Klee GG. Four-marker serum screening for Down's syndrome. *Prenat Diagn.* 1994 Aug;14(8):707–716.

Wald NJ, Hackshaw AK. Combining ultrasound and biochemistry in first-trimester screening for Down's syndrome. *Prenat Diagn.* 1997 Sep;17(9):821–829.

Wald NJ. Guidance on terminology. *J Med Screen.* 2008;15(1):50.

Wald NJ, Rish S, Hackshaw AK. Combining nuchal translucency and serum markers in prenatal screening for Down syndrome in twin pregnancies. *Prenat Diagn.* 2003;23(7):5880592.

Wang E, Batey A, Struble C. Gestational age and maternal weight effects on fetal cell-free DNA in maternal plasma. *Prenat Diagn.* 2013;33:662.

Wang L, Meng Q, Tang X, Yin T, Zhang J, Yang S, Wang X, Wu H, Shi Q, Jenkins EC, Zhong N, Gu Y. Maternal mosaicism of sex chromosome causes discordant sex chromosomal aneuploidies associated with noninvasive prenatal testing. *Taiwan J Obstet Gynecol.* 2015 Oct;54(5):527–531.

Wang Y, Chen Y, Tian F, Zhang J, Song Z, Wu Y, Han X, Hu W, Ma D, Cram D, Cheng W. Maternal mosaicism is a significant contributor to discordant sex chromosomal aneuploidies associated with noninvasive prenatal testing. *Clin Chem.* 2014 Jan;60(1):251–259.

Woodward, Kennedy, Sohaet. *Diagnostic Imaging Obstetrics*. 3rd Ed. Philadelphia: Elsevier; 2016. pp. 883–915.

Yu SC, Lee SW, Jiang P, Leung TY, Chan KC, Chiu RW, Lo YM. High-resolution profiling of fetal DNA clearance from maternal plasma by massively parallel sequencing. *Clin Chem*. 2013 Aug;59(8):1228–1237.

4

Prenatal Diagnosis

Prenatal diagnosis is the term used to describe a set of tests that are designed to determine whether a specific genetic condition is present in a fetus. This is in contrast to screening (described in Chapter 3), where the test is designed to determine if a fetus is at increased risk of having a specific genetic condition. The objective of prenatal diagnosis is to provide the patient and the OB care provider with enough information about a particular health problem to make a fully informed decision regarding pregnancy management (American College of Obstetricians and Gynecologists [ACOG], 2016).

Techniques

There are two types of procedures that can be performed for a prenatal diagnosis: *chorionic villus sampling* (CVS) and *amniocentesis*. These procedures are often referred to as *invasive testing methods* as they require a needle to be inserted either transabdominally (through the abdomen) or transcervically (through the cervix) to obtain the sample for testing. Prenatal diagnosis cannot be performed with only the use of maternal blood. Both CVS and amniocentesis are performed using ultrasound guidance. An ultrasound prior to and during the procedures evaluates for fetal viability as well as positioning (Rhoades, 1989). Both procedures have a sensitivity that approaches 100% (Simpson, 2012).

Chorionic Villus Sampling

CVS is the only diagnostic testing procedure available in the first trimester of pregnancy. This technique involves the collection of tissue, the chorionic villi, from the placenta using a needle inserted either transcervically or transabdominally. The type of CVS performed often depends on patient and provider preference, but clinical information may dictate which is the most appropriate (Alfirevic et al., 2003; Eisenberg, Wapner, 2002). CVS is commonly called a *placental biopsy*. The chorionic villi are small finger-like outgrowths of the placental tissue that develop to maximize the surface area that comes in contact with maternal blood. The fetus and the placenta arise from the same cells and thus typically have the same genetic makeup (Rhoades, 1989). The chorionic villi tissue is then sent to a laboratory to perform genetic testing.

CVS is typically performed between 10w0d and 13w6d by last menstrual period (LMP) dating. This window of time is used to minimize the risks associated with the procedure but also to allow time for the laboratory results to be obtained in the first trimester (Eisenberg, Wapner, 2002). CVS may be performed outside of this gestational age window in special circumstances, such as in the presence of oligohydramnios in the second trimester, when an amniocentesis would typically be performed (Podobnik et al., 1997).

Twins

The CVS procedure in twins may differ depending on the chorionicity of the gestation (refer to Chapter 1 for explanation of chorionicity). Chorionicity, location of the fetuses, and location of the placentas must be determined prior to undergoing a CVS procedure. These must be documented extremely well to determine which fetus each test result belongs to (Weisz, 2005). In dichorionic twin pregnancies, each fetus will likely have a unique test result, whereas in a monochorionic twin pregnancy the fetuses are typically identical, although cases have been reported where monochorionic fetuses had discordant genetic results (Dallapiccola et al., 1985; Perlman et al., 1990; Rogers et al., 1982). Both transabdominal and transcervical procedures can be performed in twin pregnancies and in fact may both be done on the same pregnancy if the location of the placentas allows for better sampling that way (Vink et al., 2012; Weisz, 2005).

Twin-twin contamination is a complication associated with CVS in twin pregnancies (Wapner, 1993). This is when the sample from one twin gets mixed in with a sample from the second twin. This can result in unclear or incorrect test results. When chorionicity cannot be determined or the placentas are fused, the tissue sample should be taken furthest away from the site of fusion to avoid sampling the same placenta twice. When this is difficult, taking a sample closer to the site of umbilical cord insertion may also reduce contamination (Weisz, 2005). When there are two amniotic sacs, special care should be taken to not pass through one sac to get to the other if at all possible. When this is not possible, every effort should be made to only remove a tissue sample from the desired placenta. Fetal sex may be used to rule out contamination in half of twin procedures (Weisz, 2005). If there is uncertainty in the CVS test results in twin pregnancies, it may be recommended that the results be confirmed with an amniocentesis (Vink et al., 2012).

Risks

CVS has been demonstrated to be highly safe; however, as with any medical procedure there are risks associated with performing the procedure. One of the most significant risks for an invasive diagnostic test such as CVS is the risk of fetal loss. The background risk for first-trimester miscarriage is higher than in subsequent trimesters, which can make it more difficult to determine which losses were due directly to the CVS procedure and which were spontaneous. It is generally accepted that the risk of fetal loss with a CVS is between 1/500 and 1/300 (0.2% and 0.3%) (ACOG, 2016; Akolekar et al., 2015; Brambati, Tului, 2005; Mujezinovic, 2007). The range is reported to be inversely related to the experience of the person or clinic who performs the procedure (Brambati, 2005; Eisenberg, Wapner, 2002). The risk of pregnancy loss after CVS in a dichorionic twin pregnancy is thought to be increased over that of singleton pregnancies. Though difficult to calculate specific procedure-related risk, it is estimated that between 1% and 4% of twin pregnancies will be lost after CVS (Agarwal, Alfirevic, 2012; Vink et al., 2012; Weisz, 2005). There have not been enough studies to provide a risk specific to monochorionic twin pregnancies (Vink et al., 2012; Weisz, 2005). Risk factors for increased risk of pregnancy loss after CVS include operator inexperience, small-for-gestational-age fetus, and more than three needle insertions (Vink et al., 2012; Wapner, 1993).

Limb reduction is a risk that is often quoted as being related to CVS. Limb reduction occurs when a portion of or the entire arm or leg does not form completely or at all. These anomalies were raised as a concern after CVS when two groups reported an increase in the incidence of limb reduction after a CVS procedure. Limb reduction anomalies are relatively rare as spontaneous defects. When this finding was evaluated further, it was found that all of the CVSs that were performed and resulted in a fetus with a limb reduction anomaly were performed earlier than 9 weeks' gestation by LMP. In subsequent studies where CVS was performed between 10 and 13 weeks by LMP, limb reduction anomalies were not found to be a statistically significant risk (Bianchi et al., 2000; Brambati, Tului, 2005; Eisenberg, Wapner, 2002; Wilson, 2000). Therefore it is not recommended that CVS be performed earlier than 10 weeks except in very exceptional circumstances, and, even then, the patient must be informed of the risk of limb reduction related to the procedure (Eisenberg, Wapner 2002; Wilson, 2000).

Other risks related to CVS include bleeding, cramping, tenderness at the needle insertion site, fluid leak, and infection (Bianchi et al., 2000; Eisenberg, Wapner, 2002; Stone, 1993). Maternal–fetal hemorrhage has also been reported (Eisenberg, Wapner, 2002). Hemangiomas have been observed in infants after a CVS procedure (Burton et al., 1995).

Limitations

Aside from the risks of the procedure itself, there are limitations to CVS. Confined placental mosaicism is a well-recognized drawback of CVS. Mosaicism is the presence of two cell lines with different chromosomal complements within the same individual (Jenkins, Wapner, 1999). Mosaicism can occur only in the placenta (confined placental mosaicism), only in the fetus (confined fetal mosaicism), or in both placenta and fetus. Mosaicism is detected in 1–2% of CVS tissue samples; however, mosaicism is only confirmed to also be present in the fetus 10–40% of the time. This means that a large percentage of the time when mosaicism is detected in a CVS sample it is confined to the placenta and not reflective of fetal genetics (Eisenberg, Wapner, 2002; Hahnemann, Vejerslev, 1997; Wapner, 2005; Wilson, 2000). Though it is rare, this can cause the results of a laboratory test done on a CVS sample to be incorrect (i.e., false positive or false negative) (Eisenberg, Wapner, 2002; Hahnemann, Vejerslev, 1997). Thus, any incidence of mosaicism in a CVS sample should be followed-up with additional testing, such as amniocentesis or fetal blood sampling (Schreck et al., 1990).

Trisomy rescue is a common cause of placental mosaicism. This phenomenon occurs when a trisomy has occurred at conception and the fertilized ovum "rescues" itself by losing one of the extra chromosomes at random so that only two remain, and the fertilized ovum is now diploid (Wapner, 2005). The remaining two chromosomes can be from either parent in any combination. For example, there could be one chromosome from each parent, or the two chromosomes could be from the same parent (called *uniparental disomy*). There is a theoretical 1 in 3 chance for any scenario (Eisenberg, Wapner, 2002). Uniparental disomy inheritance of certain chromosomes can lead to very specific genetic conditions in a baby after birth, such as Angelman syndrome and Prader-Willi syndrome. When mosaicism of certain chromosomes, such as 15, is detected in a CVS sample, it is important to consider trisomy rescue as a mechanism and assess the fetus for uniparental disomy. Follow-up is recommended when other chromosomes that are imprinted—7, 11, 14, and 22—are found to be trisomic or mosaic in a CVS sample (Eisenberg, Wapner, 2002; Ledbetter, Engel, 1995; Wapner, 2005).

Contamination is a risk that is associated with any medical and/ or lab procedure. *Maternal cell contamination* refers to the presence of maternal cells in the tissue sample obtained from the placenta. The risk of maternal cell contamination is that the genetic laboratory results obtained from the CVS sample could be from the maternal cells and not the villi from the placenta that represents the fetus. This could result in false-negative results as the mother most likely does not have a genetic condition. Testing can be performed to rule out maternal cell contamination with the use of a maternal blood sample analyzed alongside the placental tissue (Eisenberg, Wapner, 2002).

Last, there are limitations to the type of testing that can be performed on a CVS tissue sample. These include testing for open neural tube defects (ONTDs), imprinting disorders or methylation defects, and some biochemical testing. Please see the later section on "Testing Options" for a complete discussion.

Amniocentesis

An amniocentesis is a similar procedure to a CVS in that a sample of cells is collected for genetic testing. This technique involves collecting a sample of amniotic fluid through a needle inserted transabdominally. Amniotic fluid is liquid that surrounds the fetus during pregnancy and is made up primarily of fetal urine and pulmonary fluids. Amniotic fluid is important for fetal growth, nutrition, and protection (Underwood et al., 2005). Since mainly the fetus produces this fluid, it comprises fetal cells that can be used for genetic testing. Amniocentesis and amniotic fluid may be used for other types of obstetric testing, such as fetal lung maturity, or for other concerns, such as polyhydramnios fluid reduction. An amniocentesis for the purpose of genetic testing is sometimes called a *genetic amniocentesis* (Vink et al., 2012).

Amniocentesis is typically performed between 15w0d and 18w6d weeks by LMP. Confirmation of fusion between the amnion and chorion is typically the first criteria for determining when a person can have an amniocentesis. This typically occurs around 15–16 weeks. An amniocentesis may be performed later in gestation for various reasons (O'Donoghue et al., 2007; Picone et al., 2008; Vink et al., 2012). The American College of Obstetricians and Gynecologists (ACOG) states that amniocentesis before 13–14 weeks gestation (early amniocentesis) should not be carried out for genetic indications due to the increase in fetal risks (ACOG, 2016).

Twins

Amniocentesis can also be performed in twin pregnancies. Just as in CVS, the determination of chorionicity is important prior to obtaining a sample. In monochorionic twins, the procedure is the same as in a singleton pregnancy: only a single needle insertion and withdrawal of one fluid sample is necessary. As long as the fetuses are concordant for growth and anatomy it is assumed that the fetuses are genetically identical (Audibert, 2011; Weisz, 2005). Typically, in a dichorionic twin pregnancy, two needle insertions are required. After the first needle has withdrawn the necessary amount of fluid, a small amount of a blue dye called indigo carmine is injected into the sac of the first twin. This allows the operator to know if he/she has sampled the same fluid twice. Then the needle is placed into the sac of the second twin and fluid is withdrawn (Vink et al., 2012; Weisz, 2005). A second method of amniocentesis in twin pregnancies is the *single-needle technique*. This method involves the insertion of the needle into the sac of one twin, withdrawing the fluid, and then attaching a new syringe while the needle remains inside the amniotic sac. The needle is then pushed through the septum that divides the two amniotic cavities and into the second sac, where fluid is then withdrawn. The risk with the single-needle method is contamination from the first sac (Vink et al., 2012; Weisz, 2005).

Risks

As in CVS, amniocentesis has a risk of pregnancy loss associated with the procedure. The ACOG states a risk of pregnancy loss of 1/300–1/500 after amniocentesis (ACOG, 2016). In twin pregnancies, the risk for procedure-related pregnancy loss is estimated to be higher than in singleton pregnancies. Some studies report a 1% increase over the baseline risk, but the exact risk in twin pregnancies is unknown (Agarwal, Alfirevic, 2012; Akolekar et al., 2015; Enzensberger et al., 2012; Vink et al., 2012; Weisz, 2005).

As alluded to previously, there are increased risks with performing an amniocentesis prior to the recommended gestational age. These risks include elevated risk for fetal loss and a risk of clubfoot (talipes equinovarus). During the time preceding 15 weeks gestation, the two membranes of the amniotic sac have not fused. The amniotic fluid needed for genetic testing must be collected from the inner sac, and thus the needle must penetrate both membranes to obtain it, which is more technically difficult. This is associated with a statistically significant increase in the risk for pregnancy loss (Alfirevic et al., 2003; Eisenberg, Wapner, 2002). When performing an early amniocentesis, the risk for clubfoot deformity increases from 0.1% to 0.3% in the general population to about 1.5% (Eisenberg, Wapner, 2002). This is thought to be related to the increased likelihood for fluid leak after the early procedure as well as to the loss of room for proper leg movement with fluid aspiration. Fluid leakage is much less associated with CVS procedures around the same gestational age (Brambati, Tului, 2005). If a diagnostic procedure is desired during the first trimester, it is recommended that CVS be used (ACOG, 2016).

As with CVS, other risks include bleeding, cramping, tenderness at the needle insertion site, fluid leak, infection, and hemorrhage (Bianchi et al., 2000; Eisenberg, Wapner, 2002; Rhoades, 1989; Stone, Lockwood, 1993). RhoGAM is administered when a patient is Rh negative to prevent Rhesus alloimmunization and completing an amniocentesis (Eisenberg, Wapner, 2002). Some studies have indicated risks of other effects after amniocentesis, such as neonatal distress syndrome and congenital pneumonia, though this risk has not been confirmed in other studies (Eisenberg, Wapner, 2002; Tabor et al., 1986). Risk of fetal needle puncture is low with the use of ultrasound but can still occur and lead to fetal injury to the skin, eyes, chest, and cranium (Brambati, Tului, 2002; Eisenberg, Wapner, 2002).

Testing Options

Once a sample has been obtained from either CVS or amniocentesis, it is sent to a laboratory for analysis. The type of analysis performed on the sample depends on the indication for the testing as well as the specific type of information sought with the result.

There are two types of preparations that are carried out on CVS and amniotic fluid samples: cell culture and direct preparation. *Cell culture* involves taking the cells obtained from the sample and putting them in an artificial environment (outside the body) that fosters growth. The cells multiply to produce a larger number which generates enough cells to use in the testing. This process requires allowing ample time for cells to grow (Chitham et al., 1973; Keagle, Gersen, 2005). In *direct preparation*, the cells from a tissue or fluid sample can be used directly in a laboratory test without any culturing. The advantage to direct preparation is that the test results are often available more quickly than if cells were cultured first (South et al., 2008).

Karyotype

Karyotyping is one of the oldest technologies available for analyzing fetal chromosomes. Karyotyping analyzes whether there are changes in the number of chromosomes present (aneuploidy) or rearrangement of chromosomes (such as translocations or inversions), and it identifies large deletions/duplications of genetic material (typically between 3 and 10Mb in size) (Lo et al.,

2014; South et al., 2008). Karyotyping requires the use of cultured cells. Some of the cells are removed from the culture and dropped onto glass slides where they are stained and then analyzed under a microscope (Keagle, Gersen, 2005). The stain that is applied to the cells will produce a pattern of light and dark sections along each chromosome, called the *banding pattern*. Most often this is *G-banding*, where G refers to the Giemsa stain. When Giemsa is applied to the chromosomes along with trypsin, any region of the chromosome that has a high concentration of A-T bases will stain dark while any areas that are G-C rich will be seen as light bands (Keagle, Gersen, 2005). (Of note, there are other types of banding techniques that will not be discussed here.) Each chromosome pair will have a unique banding pattern. The chromosomes are then paired together based on their banding pattern, which allows the technician to determine if there are any that are missing (monosomy) or present in excess (trisomy). This process is repeated across a number of cells to be sure the result is uniform across all cells and determine if mosaicism is present. An image is then taken of one set of representative chromosomes lined up by pair and organized by size. This image is called a *karyotype* (Keagle, Gersen, 2005). An example of normal female and male karyotypes is shown in Figure 4.1, and a karyotype showing a male with trisomy 21 is shown in Figure 4.2.

Fluorescence in Situ Hybridization (FISH)

FISH is a testing method that allows for an analysis of the most common aneuploidies as well as some other chromosomal abnormalities. FISH is done by hybridizing (attaching) a DNA probe that is labeled with a specific chemical that will fluoresce under ultraviolet (UV) light (ACOG, 2014). This probe is attached at a specific location along the chromosome, such as the centromere, a unique sequence of DNA, or the whole chromosome. The chromosomes are then visualized under a microscope to analyze the presence, quantity, and/or location of the fluorescing probe (ACOG, 2014; Wolff, Schwartz, 2005). See Figure 4.3.

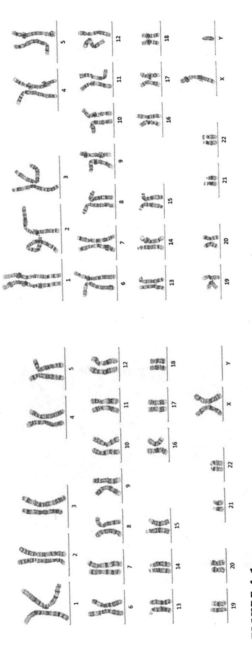

FIGURE 4.1

Normal female and male karyotypes.

Image courtesy of ARUP laboratories

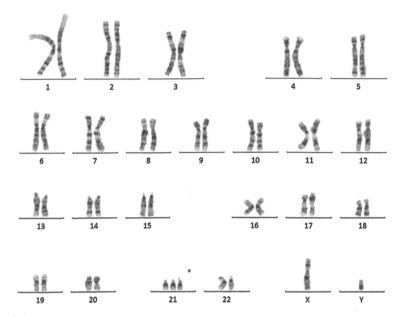

FIGURE 4.2

Male karyotype with trisomy 21.

Image courtesy of ARUP laboratories

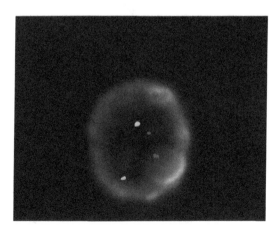

FIGURE 4.3

Normal fluorescence in situ hybridization (FISH) where bright white spots represent green probe signals and light grey spots represent red probe signals.

Image courtesy of ARUP laboratories

In the prenatal setting, visualization of the centromere of a chromosome can be used to detect aneuploidy. A typical "prenatal FISH" panel includes analysis of chromosomes 21, 18, 13, X, and Y (although the technology is able to label any chromosome) (Philip et al., 1994; Wolff, Schwartz, 2005). Rapid testing is available that does not require cells to be cultured prior to testing; this is sometimes called *interphase FISH* (Philip et al., 1994). Each of these chromosomes is labeled with a probe and then visualized under the microscope. Chromosome 21 and 13 are usually analyzed together, whereas 18, X, and Y are analyzed together (Wolff, Schwartz, 2005). Labeled probes can produce differently colored fluorescence, such as green or red. The laboratory knows which chromosome was labeled with which color probe. In simplistic terms, the number of fluorescent signals are counted by the technician to determine if there is an extra or a missing chromosome. For example, under the microscope, a technician sees two green signals and three red signals. Since the technician knows that chromosome 13 was labeled with green-colored probes and 21 was labeled with red-colored probes, the cells that are being analyzed are trisomy 21. See Figure 4.4.

FISH using unique DNA probes can be also be used in the prenatal setting. This requires cultured cells and is sometimes called *metaphase FISH*. It is most often used to detect small deletions or duplications that may not be visualized by a traditional karyotype as well as the characterization of other rearrangements and marker chromosomes (ACOG, 2014; Wolff, Schwartz, 2005). Microdeletions and microduplications can be associated with syndromes due to the loss of a large number of genes that were next to each other on the chromosome. A probe can be designed to hybridize to a specific DNA sequence that is known to be located within the region of deletion or duplication, thus allowing for the visualization of the gain or loss of that sequence by the number of fluorescent probes seen under the microscope (i.e., one probe is a loss of that region).

Interphase FISH can be useful in its ability to provide rapid results; however, since the chromosomes themselves are not being analyzed, it is not recommended as a stand-alone test (ACOG,

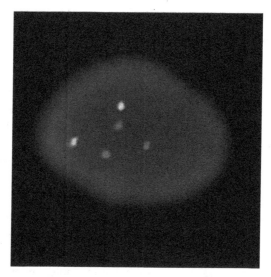

FIGURE 4.4

Abnormal fluorescence in situ hybridization (FISH) where bright white spots represent green probe signals and light grey spots represent red probe signals.

Image courtesy of ARUP laboratories

2016). Standard prenatal FISH is unable to detect chromosome rearrangements, microduplications and microdeletions, and low-level mosaicism, and it is unable to provide structural information regarding any aneuploidy detected (South et al., 2008). For example, trisomy 21 detected by FISH cannot distinguish trisomy 21 as three free chromosomes from trisomy 21 due to a Robertsonian translocation (chromosome 21 attached to chromosome 14). Positive results should be confirmed with either karyotype or microarray (see the next section) or correlated with ultrasound findings or an abnormal screening test (ACOG, 2016). FISH is not used for genome-wide assessment of the chromosomes (Lo et al., 2014).

Microarray

There are two types of microarray technology: comparative genomic hybridization and single nucleotide polymorphism

(SNP)-based technology (ACOG, 2013). Both technologies are similar and are available on fetal samples. Microarray technology is similar to FISH in that it uses probe-labeled DNA from the fetal sample and compares it to a known normal sample (ACOG, 2014). Computer software measures the difference in fluorescence and uses that information to determine if there are any gains or losses of genetic material (including trisomies), also called *copy number variants* (Schaaf et al., 2011; South et al., 2008; Wolff, Schwartz, 2005). Please see Figure 4.5 for an example of a software readout of a microarray. Because there are different technologies that provide similar information, the technology/tests are collectively called "microarray," but they may also be referred to by their more specific names including comparative genomic hybridization (CGH) array, SNP array, or simply chromosomal microarray analysis (CMA). Microarray technology can be performed on uncultured cells, allowing a more rapid analysis when compared to karyotype.

Microarray has the ability to detect small gains and losses across the entire genome of the sample that may not be detected by karyotype (as small as 100–200 kb). The ability of this technology to analyze smaller chromosomal abnormalities allows for the detection of more clinically relevant genetic conditions than karyotype alone would have detected, even in pregnancies

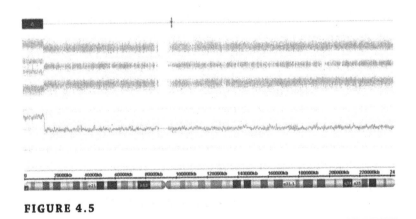

FIGURE 4.5

Microarray technology.

with a normal ultrasound (ACOG, 2016; Hillman et al., 2013; Wapner, 2012). However, because microarray technology is based on a comparison of DNA, it does not have the ability to detect balanced chromosomal rearrangements (Lo et al., 2014; Rickman et al., 2005; South et al., 2008). SNP-based technology also has the ability to detect uniparental disomy and regions of homozygosity, which are regions across the genome that are identical (typically indicating consanguinity) (ACOG, 2013; Schaaf et al., 2011; Srebniak et al., 2011; Van den Veyver et al., 2006). Microarray also has the ability to detect copy number variants that have unknown clinical significance (*variants of unknown significance [VUS]*), which means that a gain or loss of genetic material was detected in the sample, but it is unknown whether that might cause clinical symptoms or is simply due to normal variation among people (ACOG 2013; Lo et al., 2014; South et al., 2008). *Benign variants*, meaning that the gain or loss is known to not be associated with clinical symptoms, may also be detected with microarray, although these are not reported. Of note, microarray does not have the ability to detect single nucleotide or other small molecular changes.

Molecular Testing

CVS and amniotic fluid samples can be used to diagnose a fetus with known single-gene conditions including recessive, dominant, and X-linked conditions (Eisenberg, Wapner, 2002). For prenatal molecular testing, it is often required that the parental mutation(s) be known prior to pursuing a fetal diagnosis (South et al., 2008). For recessive conditions, both parents' mutations must be known; for X-linked conditions, the maternal mutation must be known; and in inherited dominant conditions, the mutation of the affected parent must be known. Dominant conditions can be the exception to this requirement when it is thought that the mutation is *de novo* in the fetus. Typically, in these cases, an ultrasound finding is the indication for pursuing testing of that particular condition (ACOG, 2014).

AFP and AChE

Amniotic fluid samples, but not CVS, can be used to diagnose ONTDs. Alpha-fetoprotein (AFP) is measured in the amniotic fluid, just as in maternal serum screening (see Chapter 3). If the AFP is also elevated in the amniotic fluid, a secondary measurement is taken of a chemical called *acetylcholinesterase (AChE)*. AChE is primarily found in the central nervous system. It is not normally found in amniotic fluid unless there is an opening along the fetal neural tube that allows it to seep out. When AChE is present in conjunction with elevated AFP in amniotic fluid, it is considered diagnostic for an ONTD (Cheschier et al., 2003). Abnormal results are generally followed by ultrasound to visualize the extent and location of the defect.

Other Testing

There are many other types of laboratory tests that are available using CVS or amniocentesis samples that are too great in number to discuss thoroughly in this text. Some tests are more useful for general obstetric care, such as Rh antigen genotyping. Others are useful for diagnosing genetic conditions but have special requirements for testing such as peroxisomal, biochemical, or methylation conditions. For most tests, analysis can be performed using either CVS or amniocentesis samples; however, this is not universally true. Some laboratory tests can only be performed on amniocytes and others only on chorionic villi (Eisenberg, Wapner, 2002). For example, methylation testing is typically not recommended on a CVS sample because the methylation pattern has not yet been set in chorionic villi, such as in fragile-X. While chorionic villi could provide information on the repeat sizes in a fragile-X case, the methylation pattern might not be clear. To confirm methylation, amniocentesis would be needed (Finucane et al., 2012; McConkie-Rosell et al., 2005). Another example is when a familial mutation cannot be identified for osteogenesis imperfecta; in this case, a CVS sample may be used to measure collagen production to make a prenatal diagnosis (Cohn, Byers, 1990; Pepin et al., 1997). It is important for genetic counselors to educate themselves and verify all laboratory testing requirements prior to offering a prenatal diagnostic test to a patient. This includes knowing which laboratory testing is available, the types of samples that can be used, whether culturing of the sample is needed, what type of collection vessel is required, sample storage and handling requirements, and laboratory send-out procedures.

Indications for Diagnostic Testing

Indications for diagnostic testing include maternal age of 35 or older, abnormal prenatal screening result from maternal serum screening or cfDNA, a woman with a previous child or pregnancy affected by a genetic condition, an anomaly identified on ultrasound, increased risk for a single-gene condition, and a parent with a known chromosome rearrangement. However, the ACOG states that "all pregnant women should be offered prenatal assessment for aneuploidy by screening or diagnostic testing regardless of maternal age or other risk factors" (ACOG, 2016).

The type of laboratory testing elected after a diagnostic procedure depends on the indication. The ACOG states that

[C]hromosomal microarray analysis has been found to detect a pathogenic (or likely pathogenic) copy number variant in approximately 1.7% of patients with a normal ultrasound examination result and a normal karyotype, and it is recommended that chromosomal microarray analysis be made available to any patient choosing to undergo invasive diagnostic testing. . . . When structural abnormalities are detected by prenatal ultrasound examination, chromosomal microarray will identify clinically significant chromosomal abnormalities in approximately 6% of the fetuses that have a normal karyotype. For this reason, chromosomal microarray analysis should be recommended as the primary test (replacing conventional karyotype) for patients undergoing prenatal diagnosis for the indication of a fetal structural abnormality detected by ultrasound examination. If a structural abnormality is strongly suggestive of a particular aneuploidy in the fetus (eg, duodenal atresia or an atrioventricular heart defect, which are characteristic of trisomy 21), karyotype with or without FISH may be offered before chromosomal microarray analysis. (ACOG, 2016)

Conclusion

A perinatal genetic counselor is an expert when it comes to knowledge of prenatal diagnosis. A patient deciding whether prenatal diagnosis is the right choice for them will have many questions, which may include anything from the steps of the procedure and its associated risks to the specific tests available and what information test results will give them. A perinatal genetic counselor must be prepared to navigate these questions and provide accurate information relevant to the current situation. Additionally, a perinatal genetic counselor is often seen as the expert on prenatal diagnosis among other providers and should be prepared to make recommendations for test utility in various situations and to have up-to-date knowledge of professional guidelines and recommendations.

References

Agarwal K, Alfirevic Z. Pregnancy loss after chorionic villus sampling and genetic amniocentesis in twin pregnancies: a systematic review. *Ultrasound Obstet Gynecol.* 2012 Aug;40(2):128–134.

Akolekar R, Beta J, Picciarelli G, Ogilvie C, D'Antonio F. Procedure-related risk of miscarriage following amniocentesis and chorionic villus sampling: a systematic review and meta-analysis. *Ultrasound Obstet Gynecol.* 2015 Jan;45(1):16–26.

Alfirevic Z, Sundberg K, Brigham S. Amniocentesis and chorionic villus sampling for prenatal diagnosis. *Cochrane Database Syst Rev.* 2003;(3):CD003252.

American College of Obstetricians and Gynecologists. Technology Assessment No. 11: Genetics and molecular diagnostic testing. *Obstet Gynecol.* 2014 Feb;123(2 Pt 1):394–413.

American College of Obstetricians and Gynecologists Committee on Genetics. Committee Opinion no. 581: the use of chromosomal microarray analysis in prenatal diagnosis. *Obstet Gynecol.* 2013 Dec;122(6):1374–1377.

American College of Obstetricians and Gynecologists Practice Bulletin no. 162 Summary: Prenatal diagnostic testing for genetic disorders. *Obstet Gynecol.* 2016 May;127(5):976–978.

Audibert F, Gagnon A. Prenatal screening for and diagnosis of aneuploidy in twin pregnancies. *J Obstet Gynaecol Can.* 2011 Jul;33(7):754–767.

Dallapiccola B, Stomeo C, Ferranti G. Discordant sex in one of three monozygotic triplets. *J Med Genet.* 1985;22:6–11.

Bianchi DW, Crombleholme TM, D'Alton ME. Fetology: diagnosis and management of the fetal patient. New York: McGraw-Hill;2000.

Brambati B, Tului L. Chorionic villus sampling and amniocentesis. *Curr Opin Obstet Gynecol.* 2005 Apr;17(2):197–201.

Burton BK, Schulz CJ, Angle B, Burd LI. An increased incidence of haemangiomas in infants born following chorionic villus sampling (CVS). *Prenat Diagn.* 1995 Mar;15(3):209–214.

Cheschier N; ACOG Committee on Practice Bulletins-Obstetrics. ACOG practice bulletin. Neural tube defects. Number 44, July 2003. (Replaces committee opinion number 252, March 2001). *Int J Gynaecol Obstet.* 2003 Oct;83(1):123–133.

Chitham RG, Quayle SJ, Hill L. The selection of a method for the culture of cells from amniotic fluid. *J Clin Pathol.* 1973 Sep;26(9):721–723.

Cohn DH, Byers PH. Clinical screening for collagen defects in connective tissue diseases. *Clin Perinatol.* 1990 Dec;17(4):793–809.

Eisenberg B, Wapner RJ. Clinical procedures in prenatal diagnosis. *Best Pract Res Clin Obstet Gynaecol.* 2002 Oct;16(5):611–627.

Enzensberger C, Pulvermacher C, Degenhardt J, Kawacki A, Germer U, Gembruch U, Krapp M, Weichert J, Axt-Fliedner R. Fetal loss rate and associated risk factors after amniocentesis, chorionic villus sampling and fetal blood sampling. *Ultraschall Med.* 2012 Dec;33(7):E75–E79.

Finucane B, Abrams L, Cronister A, Archibald AD, Bennett RL, McConkie-Rosell A. Genetic counseling and testing for FMR1 gene mutations: practice guidelines of the national society of genetic counselors. *J Genet Couns.* 2012 Dec;21(6):752–760.

Hahnemann JM, Vejerslev LO. Accuracy of cytogenetic findings on chorionic villus sampling (CVS)--diagnostic consequences of CVS mosaicism and non-mosaic discrepancy in centres contributing to EUCROMIC 1986–1992. *Prenat Diagn.* 1997 Sep;17(9):801–820.

Hillman SC, McMullan DJ, Hall G, Togneri FS, James N, Maher EJ, Meller CH, Williams D, Wapner RJ, Maher ER, Kilby MD. Use of prenatal chromosomal microarray: prospective cohort study and systematic review and meta-analysis. *Ultrasound Obstet Gynecol.* 2013 Jun;41(6):610–620.

Jenkins, T, Wapner, R. First trimester prenatal diagnosis: chorionic villus sampling. *Semin Perinatol.* 1999 Oct;23(5):403–413.

Keagle MB, Gersen SL. Basic laboratory procedures. In: Gersen SL, Keagle MB, eds. *The principles of clinical cytogenetics.* Totowa, NJ: Humana Press;2005:63–80.

Ledbetter D, Engel E. Uniparental disomy in humans: development of an imprinting map and its implications for prenatal diagnosis. *Human Mol Gen.* 1995;4:1757–1764.

Lo JO, Shaffer BL, Feist CD, Caughey AB. Chromosomal microarray analysis and prenatal diagnosis. *Obstet Gynecol Surv.* 2014 Oct;69(10):613–621.

McConkie-Rosell A, Finucane B, Cronister A, Abrams L, Bennett RL, Pettersen BJ. Genetic counseling for fragile x syndrome: updated recommendations of the national society of genetic counselors. *J Genet Couns.* 2005 Aug;14(4):249–270.

Mujezinovic F, Alfirevic Z. Procedure-related complications of amniocentesis and chorionic villous sampling: a systematic review. *Obstet Gynecol.* 2007 Sep;110(3):687–694.

O'Donoghue K, Giorgi L, Pontello V, Pasquini L, Kumar S. Amniocentesis in the third trimester of pregnancy. *Prenat Diagn.* 2007 Nov;27(11):1000–1004.

Pepin M, Atkinson M, Starman B, Byers P. Strategies and outcomes of prenatal diagnosis for osteogenesis imperfecta: a review of biochemical and molecular studies completed in 129 pregnancies. *Prenatal Diagnosis.* 1997;17:559–570.

Perlman E, Stetten G, Tuck-Muller C. Sexual discordance in monozygotic twins. *Am J Obstet Gynecol.* 1990;37:551–557.

Philip J, Bryndorf T, Christensen B. Prenatal aneuploidy detection in interphase cells by fluorescence in situ hybridization (FISH). *Prenat Diagn.* 1994 Dec;14(13):1203–1215.

Picone O, Senat MV, Rosenblatt J, Audibert F, Tachdjian G, Frydman R. Fear of pregnancy loss and fetal karyotyping: a place for third-trimester amniocentesis? *Fetal Diagn Ther.* 2008;23(1):30–35.

Podobnik M, Ciglar S, Singer Z, Podobnik-Sarkanji S, Duic Z, Skalak D. Transabdominal chorionic villus sampling in the second and third trimesters of high-risk pregnancies. *Prenat Diagn.* 1997 Feb;17(2):125–133.

Rhoads GG, Jackson LG, Schlesselman SE, de la Cruz FF, Desnick RJ, Golbus MS, et al. The safety and efficacy of chorionic villus sampling for early prenatal diagnosis of cytogenetic abnormalities. *N Engl J Med.* 1989 Mar 9;320(10):609–617.

Rickman L, Fiegler H, Carter NP, Bobrow M. Prenatal diagnosis by array-CGH. *Eur J Med Genet.* 2005 Jul-Sep;48(3):232–340.

Rogers JG, Voullaire L, Gold H. Monozygotic twins discordant for trisomy 21. *Am J Med Genet.* 1982;11:143–146.

Schaaf CP, Wiszniewska J, Beaudet, AL. Copy number and SNP arrays in clinical diagnostics. *Annu Rev Genomics Hum Genet.* 2011;12:25–51.

Schreck RR, Falik-Borenstein Z, Hirata G. Chromosomal mosaicism in chorionic villus sampling. *Clin Perinatol.* 1990 Dec;17(4):867–888.

Simpson JL. Invasive procedures for prenatal diagnosis: any future left? *Best Pract Res Clin Obstet Gynaecol.* 2012 Oct;26(5):625–638.

South ST, Chen Z, Brothman AR. Genomic medicine in prenatal diagnosis. *Clin Obstet Gynecol.* 2008 Mar;51(1):62–73.

Srebniak M, Boter M, Oudesluijs G, Joosten M, Govaerts L, Van Opstal D, Galjaard RJ. Application of SNP array for rapid prenatal diagnosis: implementation, genetic counselling and diagnostic flow. *Eur J Hum Genet.* 2011 Dec;19(12):1230–1237.

Stone JL, Lockwood CJ. Amniocentesis and chorionic villus sampling. *Curr Opin Obstet Gynecol.* 1993 Apr;5(2):211–217.

Tabor A, Philip J, Madsen U. Randomized controlled trial of genetic amniocentesis in 4606 low-risk women. *Lancet.* 1986;i:1287.

Underwood MA, Gilbert WM, Sherman MP. Amniotic fluid: not just fetal urine anymore. *J Perinatol*. 2005 May;25(5):341–348.

Van den Veyver IB, Beaudet AL. Comparative genomic hybridization and prenatal diagnosis. *Curr Opin Obstet Gynecol*. 2006 Apr;18(2):185–191.

Vink J, Wapner R, D'Alton ME. Prenatal diagnosis in twin gestations. *Semin Perinatol*. 2012 Jun;36(3):169–174.

Wapner RJ, Johnson A, Davis G, Urban A, Morgan P, Jackson L. Prenatal diagnosis in twin gestations: a comparison between second-trimester amniocentesis and first-trimester chorionic villus sampling. *Obstet Gynecol*. 1993 Jul;82(1):49–56.

Wapner RJ. Invasive prenatal diagnostic techniques. *Semin Perinatol*. 2005 Dec;29(6):401–404.

Wapner RJ, Martin CL, Levy B, Ballif BC, Eng CM, Zachary JM, et al. Chromosomal microarray versus karyotyping for prenatal diagnosis. *N Engl J Med*. 2012 Dec 6;367(23):2175–2184.

Weisz B, Rodeck C. Invasive diagnostic procedures in twin pregnancies. *Prenat Diagn*. 2005;25:751–758.

Wilson RD. Amniocentesis and chorionic villus sampling. *Curr Opin Obstet Gynecol*. 2000 Apr;12(2):81–86.

Wolff DJ, Schwartz S. Fluorescence in situ hybridization. In: Gersen SL, Keagle MB, eds. The principles of clinical cytogenetics. Totowa, NJ: Humana Press; 2005:455–489.

5

Common Indications

Individuals and families may be referred to a perinatal genetic counselor for a variety of reasons. Some of the most common indications for referral will be discussed in this chapter and include age-related risks, personal and family history, ultrasound anomalies, teratogen exposure, recurrent pregnancy loss, and preconception counseling.

Age-Related Risks

Maternal Age

One of the most common referrals to a perinatal genetic counselor is a maternal age of 35 years or older. This is often referred to as *advanced maternal age* (AMA). The frequency of this referral is likely due to the fact that women and men are having children at later ages than they were even 30 years ago (Barclay, 2016). AMA is associated with an increased risk of obstetric complications such as hypertension and preeclampsia, gestational diabetes, preterm birth, stillbirth, and multiples, as well as a decrease in overall fertility (ACOG FAQ060; Hansen, 1986; Liu, Case, 2011). In addition to these risks is the increased risk of aneuploidy with increasing maternal age (American College of Obstetricians and Gynecologists and Society for Maternal-Fetal Medicine, 2016; Hassold, Hunt, 2001; Hassold et al., 2007; Hook, 1981; Snijders et al., 1995). Of note, the risk for aneuploidy due to parental balanced chromosomal rearrangement does not increase with increasing parental age.

Approximately 5% of all clinically recognized pregnancies are aneuploid (Hassold, Hunt, 2001), and only a fraction of those conceived with a trisomy or monosomy will be compatible with a live birth, such as in trisomy 21. The majority of these aneuploid pregnancies will result in a miscarriage, and only a small percentage will make it to term (American College of Obstetricians and Gynecologists and Society for Maternal-Fetal Medicine, 2016; Hassold, Hunt, 2001; Hook et al., 1983). This means that the likelihood of a woman giving birth to a baby with an aneuploidy will be less than the likelihood for her to conceive a baby with an aneuploidy. This likelihood can be further broken down by the age of the mother. As a woman ages, there is an increase in the chance to conceive a pregnancy with a trisomy (American College of Obstetricians and Gynecologists and Society for Maternal-Fetal Medicine, 2016; Hassold, Hunt, 2001; Hook, 1981; Hook et al., 1983; Snijders et al., 1995), although every woman, regardless of age or ethnicity, can conceive a pregnancy with an aneuploidy (American College of Obstetricians and Gynecologists and Society for Maternal-Fetal Medicine, 2016; Hassold, Hunt, 2001). Table 5.1 lists the risks based on maternal age at various points through pregnancy. Limited data exists for women beyond the age of 45 (Morris, 2003). The exception to this is monosomy X, or 45,X, where an association with maternal age does not appear to be present (Hook, 1981).

A pregnant woman who is 35 years of age at the time of delivery is defined as an AMA patient. Because the term "advanced maternal age" can be controversial given its implications of being too old to have children, many prefer simply to say "age-related risks," given the fact that a woman of any age has a chance to have a baby with an aneuploidy, not just women over the age of 35. The age of 35 or older was selected as "AMA" because in the 1970s data suggested that a woman who is 35 years old has the same chance of delivering a baby with an aneuploidy as her chance of miscarriage if she completed an amniocentesis (Berkowitz, 2006). At that time, the age of 35 was used as the basis to determine who was offered prenatal testing. In essence, age was the first prenatal

TABLE 5.1 Rates of aneuploidy at term/birth and 10 weeks by maternal age

Maternal Age	Risk for Any Aneuploidy at Term[a]	Risk for Trisomy 21 at 10 Weeks[b]	Risk for Trisomy 21 at Term[a]	Risk for Trisomy 18 at 10 Weeks[b]	Risk for Trisomy 18 at Term[b]	Risk for Trisomy 18 at 10 Weeks[b]	Risk for Trisomy 13 at Term[b]
15	1/454		1/1,578				
16	1/475		1/1,572				
17	1/499		1/1,565				
18	1/525		1/1,556				
19	1/555		1/1,544				
20	1/525	1/804	1/1,480	1/1,993	1/18,013	1/6,347	1/42,423
21	1/525	1/793	1/1,460	1/1,968	1/17,782	1/6,266	1/41,878
22	1/499	1/780	1/1,440	1/1,934	1/17,479	1/6,159	1/41,165
23	1/475	1/762	1/1,420	1/1,891	1/17,086	1/3,021	1/40,241
24	1/475	1/740	1/1,380	1/1,835	1/16,584	1/5,844	1/39,057
25	1/475	1/712	1/1,340	1/1,765	1/15,951	1/5,621	1/37,567
26	1/475	1/677	1/1,290	1/1,679	1/15,170	1/5,345	1/35,728
27	1/454	1/635	1/1,220	1/1,575	1/14,231	1/5,014	1/33,515
28	1/434	1/586	1/1,140	1/1,453	1/13,133	1/4,628	1/30,930
29	1/416	1/531	1/1,050	1/1,316	1/11,895	1/4,191	1/28,015
30	1/384	1/471	1/940	1/1,168	1/10,554	1/3,719	1/24,856
31	1/384	1/409	1/820	1/1,014	1/9,160	1/3,228	1/21,573

(continued)

TABLE 5.1 Continued

Maternal Age	Risk for Any Aneuploidy at Term[a]	Risk for Trisomy 21 at 10 Weeks[b]	Risk for Trisomy 21 at Term[a]	Risk for Trisomy 18 at 10 Weeks[b]	Risk for Trisomy 18 at Term[b]	Risk for Trisomy 18 at 10 Weeks[b]	Risk for Trisomy 13 at Term[b]
32	1/322	1/347	1/700	1/860	1/7,775	1/2,740	1/18,311
33	1/285	1/288	1/570	1/715	1/6,458	1/2,275	1/15,209
34	1/243	1/235	1/456	1/582	1/5,256	1/1,852	1/12,380
35	1/178	1/187	1/353	1/465	1/4,202	1/1,481	1/9,896
36	1/148	1/148	1/267	1/366	1/3,307	1/1,165	1/7,788
37	1/122	1/115	1/199	1/284	1/2,569	1/905	1/6,050
38	1/104	1/88	1/148	1/218	1/1,974	1/696	1/4,650
39	1/80	1/67	1/111	1/167	1/1,505	1/530	1/3,544
40	1/62	1/51	1/85	1/126	1/1,139	1/401	1/2,683
41	1/48	1/38	1/67	1/95	1/858	1/302	1/2,020
42	1/38	1/29	1/54	1/71	1/644	1/227	1/1,516
43	1/30	1/21	1/45	1/53	1/481	1/170	1/1,134
44	1/23	1/16	1/39	1/40	1/359	1/127	1/846
45	1/18		1/35				

[a] American College of Obstetricians and Gynecologists and Society for Maternal-Fetal Medicine, 2016. Excludes 47, 162

[b] Snijders, 1995; Snijders, 1999; Hook, 1981.

genetic screening tool (Berkowitz, 2006). The age used for AMA when a woman is pregnant with twins is 32 years. The age selected for AMA is different for a singleton pregnancy because each fetus carries its own individual risk for aneuploidy, thus making the pregnancy double the risk. The risk for aneuploidy in at least one fetus at a maternal age of 32 is comparable to the risk for the fetus of singleton pregnancy at the age of 35 (Meyers et al., 1997; Odido et al., 2003).

Aneuploidy has primarily been found to be caused during oogenesis, specifically by nondisjunction of the chromosomes during maternal meiosis I (MI) and occasionally meiosis II (MII) (Hassold, 2001; Hassold et al., 2007; Kurahashi et al., 2012). The timing of the nondisjunction event has been further characterized to be chromosome-specific. For example, acrocentric chromosomal nondisjunction, such as chromosome 21, is predominantly an MI event while trisomy 18 and sex chromosome trisomies are most often due to an MII error (Hassold et al., 2007). Males and females differ in the timing of meiosis I in their gametes. Females initiate MI during fetal development; then the oocyte enters a state of meiotic arrest that resumes 10–15 years later, at oocyte ovulation at the age of sexual maturity. MII is then completed after the egg has been fertilized, resulting in only one egg and three polar bodies. On the other hand, males begin MI at puberty and MII occurs in sequence directly after (Hassold, Hunt, 2001). It is thought that the arrest and reinitiation of MI in females is the cause of most maternally inherited aneuploidy, although the mechanisms are still relatively unknown. Although no definitive conclusions have been reached, research suggests that a gradual loss of the cohesin complex—the complex that keeps sister-chromatids connected during the meiotic arrest from fetus to puberty—is related to the increase in incidence of aneuploidy with age. Simply stated, the longer the oocytes are in arrest, the less effectively they will complete meiosis once they are fertilized (Kurahashi et al., 2012). Other research has shown that reduced levels of recombination or a suboptimal position during recombination may also increase the likelihood of nondisjunction (Hassold, Hunt, 2001). It may be that all of these contribute to the maternal age-related risk for nondisjunction (Hassold, Hunt, 2001).

Another unique risk that has been associated with increasing maternal age is uniparental disomy (UPD). Studies have found that the risk for maternally derived UPD increases with maternal age (Ginsburg et al., 2000; Kotzot, 2010; Robinson et al., 1996). This is likely due to *trisomy rescue* (described in Chapter 4). Given that the likelihood of trisomy increases with maternal age and that one of the major mechanisms of UPD is trisomic rescue, the risk for maternal UPD will also increase with maternal age (Kotzot, 2010).

Paternal Age

There is no clear clinically accepted definition of advanced paternal age (APA), although many ages have been proposed: the American Society of Reproductive Medicine's (ASRM) practice guidelines on sperm donation suggest an age of 40, ACMG recommends an age of 40, while the American College of Gynecologists (ACOG) gives a range of from 40 to 50 years (ACOG, 2016; Practice Committee ASRM, 2013b; Kong et al., 2012; Liu et al., 2011; Ramasamy et al., 2015; Sharma et al., 2015; Toriello et al., 2008). Increasing paternal age is associated with an increasing risk of genetic conditions caused by *de novo* gene mutations (Crow, 2000; Kong et al., 2012; Toriello et al., 2008). The base substitution rate is much higher in males than in females due to the large number of cell divisions during spermatogenesis throughout a male's life (Crow, 2000; Kong et al., 2012; Toriello et al., 2008). It is estimated that two new mutations occur each year (Kong et al., 2012). This could be due to reduced efficiency of DNA replication or DNA repair mechanisms that are expected to decrease with age (Crow, 2000). Therefore, conditions associated with base substitutions are strongly associated with increasing paternal age while those caused by point mutations and base pair deletions have a lesser association. Conditions such as achondroplasia, Pfeiffer syndrome, Crouzon syndrome, Apert syndrome, and thanatophoric dysplasia are most commonly associated with advanced paternal age (Crow, 2000; Toriello et al.,

2008). Other conditions, such as autism, bipolar disorder, and schizophrenia have also been associated with advanced paternal age (Kong et al., 2012; Sharma et al., 2015; Toriello et al., 2008). Paternal age over 50 years has also been associated with increased risk of trisomy 21 (Sharma et al., 2015).

Personal and Family History

Patients may be referred to genetic counseling when they or someone in their family has a particular condition, including in a prior child or pregnancy. There are many and varied conditions that a perinatal genetic counselor may encounter with this type of referral. Some of these may be single-gene conditions with a clear inheritance pattern, while others might be multifactorial conditions with variable expressivity and no specific inheritance pattern. Common referrals for personal or family history may include single-gene conditions in which the patient or a family member has a known diagnosis, a patient with a previous child or pregnancy with a genetic condition or birth defect, a patient born with or having a family history of a birth defect, multifactorial conditions, intellectual disability (ID), or autism, as well as consanguinity between the patient and partner. Each specific condition will entail a different discussion, but the components of the genetic counseling appointment will largely be the same (as discussed in Chapter 2). These types of referrals may occur before or after a pregnancy is conceived, although prior to conception is often preferred.

Single-Gene Conditions

Single-gene conditions are sometimes called *Mendelian conditions*. These conditions typically have a known inheritance pattern with a known gene(s), such as Duchenne muscular dystrophy (Nussbaum, 2007). Given that inheritance depends on the specific condition, the genetic counselor must have a working knowledge of the condition prior to meeting with the patient. This includes the common features and symptoms of the condition, which genes are involved with causing the condition, and what the inheritance pattern is; in addition, the ability to calculate the likelihood that the patient would have a child with that particular condition, know what testing options are available to predict if the parent is a carrier or affected with the condition, and know what testing might be available for a pregnancy if the condition might affect future children. One of the key components of this type of session is confirmation of diagnosis in either the patient or the family member with the condition and knowledge of the degree of relationship to the patient and/or the fetus. This typically requires medical/testing records from the affected individual. This will ensure that the genetic counselor is speaking about the correct condition and providing accurate risk estimates and testing options.

Aneuploidy

A personal or family history of aneuploidy, such as trisomy 21, 18, or 13 and monosomy X, is a common referral. Observational research suggests that a woman who has had a previous child with a trisomy is at an increased risk, above that of her age-related risk, to have another child with an aneuploidy (Baty, 1994; de Souza, 2009; Cereda, 2012; Uehara, 1999; Warburton, 2004). This is not limited to a recurrence of the same trisomy. Women with a previous child with any trisomy are at an increased risk for any other trisomy as well (de Souza, 2009; Warburton, 2004). This risk is present outside of those who have a parental chromosomal rearrangement, such as a balanced translocation, as these recurrence risks would be much higher. It is thought that this increased risk is due to gonadal mosaicism as well as the theory that some women may be at a higher risk for nondisjunction than other women (Uehara, 1999; Warburton, 2004). The recurrence risk for any trisomy can be up to 1% (Cereda, 2012; Sachs, 1990).

For those with a family history of a trisomy other than a previous child, there is no association with an increased risk for recurrence, unless there is a chromosomal rearrangement in the family (refer to the section on Evaluation of pregnancy loss and stillbirth for information about chromosomal rearrangements).

Multifactorial Conditions

Referral for a personal or family history of a multifactorial condition is similar to that for single-gene conditions: the structure and discussion that occurs in these genetic counseling appointments is the same. However, the main difference is that multifactorial conditions are not caused by genetic mutations alone (Nussbaum, 2007). They are typically the result of the interactions between genes and other factors including environment and other genes (Bijanzadeh, 2017; Nussbaum, 2007). This means that multifactorial conditions are often seen running in families, which is likely because families share a larger proportion of their genes (and often environment) with family members than with the rest of the population. Predicting who will be affected is much more difficult and often impossible. For example, mental health conditions and diabetes may have a genetic component to them, but not everyone in a family will develop that condition. Therefore, someone could inherit the susceptibility to develop a particular multifactorial condition, but the counselor would not be able to test them or their pregnancy to determine if they have that susceptibility. To predict the likelihood of a multifactorial condition occurring in a particular person, the counselor must rely on empirical data. Empirical data or empirical evidence is gathered by observation in the population. This can be accomplished by observing the number of affected versus unaffected individuals in a family as well as the degree of relationship (Nussbaum, 2007). Various methods for estimating the probability that a familial condition will occur in a family member are available that will not be discussed here. In general, *empirical risk* is the observed recurrence in similar families for a relative of the same degree of relationship (Nussbaum, 2007). The risk that a particular multifactorial condition will occur increases when there are more family members with that condition, the condition is more severe, and when the person with the condition is of the sex that is less commonly affected (Bijanzadeh, 2017). Empirical risk is usually expressed as a percent. For example, when a person has an uncle with bipolar disorder, the chance that this individual will also develop bipolar is about 5%; however, when the person has two parents who have bipolar disorder, that risk increases to 50–70% (Nussbaum, 2007). Empirical risk estimates may change at any given time as more data are collected. It is important to conduct a primary literature search to determine the most up-to-date risk information for multifactorial conditions.

Birth Defects

A referral for family or personal history of an isolated birth defect is very similar to referrals for other multifactorial conditions. Many isolated birth defects are sporadic and have an unknown etiology (ACOG FAQ146; Basso, 1999), but some birth defects have been known to recur in families (Lie, 1994). Birth defects can be caused by parental genetic contributions or by environmental factors such as maternal conditions like diabetes, diet, infections, and exposures to medications (ACOG FAQ146; Lie, 1994). The general risk of a major structural birth defect in any given pregnancy is estimated somewhere between 2% and 6%, or around 3% (Basso, 1999; CDC, 2008). However, this risk may be adjusted based on a personal or family history of a specific birth defect. In general, women who had a previous child with a birth defect were 2.4 times more likely to have another child with the same birth defect when conceiving with the same partner (Lie, 1994). Approximately 5% of infants born to males who had a personal history of a birth defect were also born with a birth defect, compared to 2% of males without a personal history of a birth defect (Lie, 2001). Unless a birth defect is known to be caused by a genetic syndrome (which may have recurrence risks as high as 100%), empirical data are used to determine the likelihood of having a baby with the familial birth defect (Aylsworth, 1992). See Table 5.2 for common examples.

TABLE 5.2 Empirical risk estimates for common birth defects

	General Population Risk	Empiric Recurrence Risk in a First-Degree Relative	Considerations
Cleft lip with/without cleft palate	0.1%	4–8%	Palate involvement and laterality seems to affect the risk estimate for siblings of proband.
Congenital heart defect (CHD)	1%	3–5%	The type of CHD may modify this risk estimate. The risk is for any CHD and the recurrence may be a different type of CHD.
Open neural tube defect (anencephaly/spina bifida)	0.1%	1–3%	This risk is present even with a dietary folic acid supplementation.
Clubfoot	0.1%	2–7%	Risk may be affected by the specific relationship to the proband (i.e., parent vs. sibling).

(Nussbaum, 2007; Klotz, 2010;Bijanzadeh, 2017)

Intellectual Disability, Developmental Delay, and Autism

The prevalence of ID is about 1% (Maulik, 2011). ID can be classified as *idiopathic*, meaning of no known cause, or related to a syndrome (Bijanzadeh, 2017). When a person has a family history of ID, the direction of the discussion will be based on the type of ID in the family. When ID is known to be caused by a genetic condition, the discussion will be based on the mode of inheritance and the testing available for that particular condition. When ID is idiopathic, the discussion will be similar to that of a multifactorial condition with recurrence risk in siblings reported between 3% and 14% (Crow, 1998).

Determining whether the individual in the family has a syndromic or idiopathic form of ID, developmental delay, or autism is important, and records are always the best method for proper evaluation. However, when records are unavailable, the family history can be a great tool to help accomplish this by asking questions regarding other features of the individual or family members. These can include physical features of the individual with ID, what other characteristics and/or symptoms that individual might have, or related features in family members. For example, given that fragile-X is one of the most common inherited forms of ID, the ACOG recommends that anyone with a family history of unexplained ID, developmental delay, or autism be evaluated (for fragile-X ACOG no. 691). Please refer to Chapter 6 for a more complete discussion. A genetic counselor should ask probing and directed questions regarding family members with possible symptoms of fragile-X–related disorders including premature ovarian failure and intention tremors, as well as physical attributes of the individual with ID. This allows the genetic counselor to better ascertain the likelihood of fragile-X as the cause of the unexplained ID or consider other possible causes.

Recurrence for idiopathic autism is estimated to be between 2% and 8% (Muhle, 2004). While some cases of autism are due to an underlying genetic condition such as a cytogenetic disorder, fragile-X, tuberous sclerosis, or other single-gene disorders these account for less than 10% of autism diagnoses. There is much evidence to suggest that autism is more commonly due to the interaction between genetic and nongenetic factors and is thus usually a multifactorial condition (Muhle, 2004), though the identification and number of genes involved is unclear. Epidemiological evidence also suggests that environmental exposures such as teratogens and prenatal infections may account for a few cases of autism. Of note, there is no evidence to suggest that immunizations are responsible for autism (Muhle, 2004).

Consanguinity

Consanguinity is the term used to describe couples who share at least one common ancestor (Bennett et al., 2002). Unions among related individuals are considered uncommon or even stigmatized in North American culture, but, in many other cultures, it is considered normal and even a preferred choice for marriages. Consanguinity is different from the legal determination of incest, which can include unions between nonbiologically related individuals. Incest will not be discussed in this text. Consanguineous couples are often referred to genetic counseling because their offspring are at an increased risk for recessive genetic conditions, birth defects, stillbirth, infant death, and possibly multifactorial conditions compared to the offspring of parents who are unrelated (Bennett et al., 2002; Stoltenberg et al., 1999a, 1999b). For couples who are consanguineous, the degree of relationship determines the amount of risk (i.e., the more closely they are related, the higher the risk). This is because the closer the degree of relationship, the more genes the couple is predicted to share, and thus the greater the likelihood their offspring will inherit identical copies of those deleterious genes (Bennett et al., 2002). For example, siblings are predicted to share about half (50%) of their genes, whereas first cousins are predicted to share one-eighth (12.5%) of their genes; thus, offspring from sibling unions will be identical at approximately one-quarter (25%) of their gene loci, whereas offspring of first cousins will be identical at about one-sixteenth (6.25%) of their gene loci (Bennett et al., 2002). The risk estimation for consanguineous couples is determined by the population risk plus the added factor of shared genes. For example, the baseline risk for a nonconsanguineous couple to have a baby with a birth defect is 3–4%, whereas a couple who are first cousins have an additional risk for birth defects of 1.7–2.8% (Bennett et al., 2002). Given this increased risk, counseling for couples who are consanguineous should include a risk assessment by taking a detailed family history that notes the degree of relationship and offering genetic testing and screening as appropriate. When a genetic condition is suspected in the offspring of a consanguineous couple, autosomal recessive conditions should be considered as a possible etiology (Bennett et al., 2002). Consanguinity does not increase the risk of aneuploidy (Bennett et al., 2002). Pregnancies in consanguineous couples are not treated differently from those in nonconsanguineous couples. Particular care may need to be taken to address psychosocial and cultural issues when counseling a couple who is consanguineous.

Ultrasound Anomalies

It is estimated that congenital anomalies occur in approximately 3% of live births (Martin et al., 2008) and thus represent a significant portion of the population. The goal of ultrasound is to identify congenital anomalies that may not be compatible with life, are associated with a high level of morbidity, or may benefit from or necessitate specific interventions before or after delivery. The potential of ultrasound to detect congenital malformations varies widely by studies, with a range reported of 15.0% to 100% (Bricker et al., 2000), but this varies by the type of anomaly and the experience of the provider. Although the best time to assess fetal anatomy is between 18 and 20 weeks' gestation, anomalies may be identified on any ultrasound (Fong et al., 2004; Whitworth et al.,

2015), and some findings are specific to the first trimester (e.g., nuchal translucency [NT]). Although there are too many ultrasound findings and implications to discuss in entirety, here we review common considerations and hallmark abnormalities associated with aneuploidy and other genetic conditions.

Counseling for Ultrasound Anomalies

When an ultrasound finding is identified, a patient should be notified and counseled about the implications, which will vary widely depending on the finding(s). Needless to say, this is often a challenging conversation to have, and patients may have a difficult time processing all or any of the information presented. Patients may need referrals to specialists, additional counseling, or followup after the initial appointment. Key components to include in the discussion are a detailed explanation of the finding, the degree of certainty of the finding, the severity of the condition, the differential diagnoses being considered and likelihoods of these, the suspected prognosis, testing available, management options, referrals, and reproductive options.

Classification of Ultrasound Findings

Congenital anomalies can occur in isolation or in combination with multiple findings. An ultrasound finding may be due to an underlying syndrome (e.g., chromosomal, Mendelian, teratogen) or have an unknown etiology and be instead a combination of genetic and environmental factors (multifactorial). Findings are classified as either major or minor. *Major anomalies* are defined as ones that create a serious adverse effect on health and development, will require surgical or medical interventions, or result in significant cosmetic impact (e.g., spina bifida, congenital heart defects, and cleft lip). Conversely, *minor anomalies* are findings that do not cause a significant impact on morbidity. Minor anomalies on ultrasound are often termed *"soft markers"*, or "findings of uncertain significance", meaning that they are often normal variants with no clinical consequences but are associated with an increased risk of fetal abnormality. Keep in mind that some findings may initially be considered soft markers but have the potential to progress to major anomalies requiring follow-up (e.g., urinary tract dilation, ventriculomegaly, and echogenic bowel).

Estimating Risks

Ultrasound has a critical role in the identification of chromosome abnormalities, genetic conditions, and birth defects, however, ultrasound is not diagnostic of these conditions nor is a normal ultrasound a guarantee of a healthy baby. Rather, it can be considered as another screening tool, and, therefore, information from the ultrasound can be combined with other factors (e.g., maternal age, screening results, family history) to give more specific risk estimates. When a structural anomaly or anomalies are identified, determination of the percentage of cases that are expected to have aneuploidy or another genetic condition is helpful for counseling. For example, an atrioventricular septal defect detected prenatally has a reported 50% chance that the fetus will have Down syndrome (Morlando et al., 2017). Similarly, when a soft marker is identified, a new risk can be calculated using the reported likelihood ratios (LR). To do this, one simply multiplies the LR and the *a priori* risk (starting risk). For example, a patient with an age-related risk of 1 in 1,000 for Down syndrome identified with an increased nuchal fold, which has a positive LR of 23.3 (Agathokleous et al., 2013), would then have a 23.3 in 1,000 (1 in 43) risk. Negative likelihood ratios, given the absence of findings, can also be used in the same manner to show reduced risks.

Ultrasound Findings in Pregnancies with Aneuploidy

Here we review major and minor findings (soft markers) of the most common chromosomal aneuploidies, including trisomies 21,

18, and 13; Turner syndrome; and triploidy as well as review other common ultrasound findings and their implications.

Down Syndrome

The prevalence of Down syndrome is approximately 1 in 600, including live births, stillbirths, and terminations (Parker et al., 2010). Multiple structural anomalies have been observed in fetuses with Down syndrome. Approximately 30% will have a major structural anomaly present, and about 50–60% will have one or more findings, including soft markers, seen on an 18- to 20-week anatomy scan (Papp et al., 2008). The most common major structural anomalies include cardiac defects (ventricular septal defect, atrioventricular septal defect, and tetralogy of Fallot), duodenal atresia, cystic hygroma, and moderate to severe ventriculomegaly (>12 mm). Soft markers can be identified in the first or second trimester. The first-trimester markers include increased NT (>3.0 mm), absent or hypoplastic nasal bone, and abnormal ductus venosus flow. Generally recognized second-trimester markers are increased nuchal fold (≥6 mm), absent or hypoplastic nasal bone, echogenic bowel, echogenic intracardiac focus, urinary tract dilation, short long bones (humerus or femur), echogenic bowel, and mild ventriculomegaly (10–12 mm). Additional soft markers may include unfused amnion and chorion after 16 weeks of pregnancy, sandal gap foot, and fifth-finger clinodactyly (Woodward et al., 2016). See Table 5.3 for a list of second-trimester soft markers associated with Down syndrome, a description, and available reported likelihood ratios.

Trisomy 18

Trisomy 18 occurs in approximately 1 in 3,000 live births, stillbirths, and terminations in the United States (Parker et al., 2010). Fetuses with trisomy 18 often have one or more major or minor findings identified on an 18- to 20-week anatomy ultrasound. Studies vary on the reported sensitivity of ultrasound to detect trisomy 18, with

TABLE 5.3 Second-trimester soft markers associated with Down syndrome and likelihood ratios

Soft Marker	Description	Likelihood Ratio
Intracardiac echogenic focus	A bright spot or area of echogenicity typically found within the ventricles of the fetal heart in the region of the papillary muscle or chordae tendineae. This is thought to represent mineralization, or small deposits of calcium, in the muscle of the heart. In high-risk patients, studies suggest an association with an increased risk of aneuploidy. This is considered a benign finding in low-risk populations.	5.08–5.83
Urinary tract dilation (UTD) mild (previously known as pelviectasis, pyelectasis, fetal hydronephrosis)	Increased anterior-posterior renal pelvis diameter (AP RPD). Stratified into mild (UTD A1) or severe (UTD A2–3). Normal AP RPD measurements are <4 mm from 16–27 weeks and <7 mm when ≥28 weeks. UTD A1 is 4 to <7 mm at <28 weeks and 7 to <10 mm at ≥28 weeks. UTD A2–3 is >7 mm at <28 weeks and >10 mm ≥28 weeks. If UTD A1 is identified, a follow-up ultrasound at ≥32 weeks and two ultrasound after birth at >48 hours to 1 month and 1–6 months later is recommended. If UTD A2–3 is identified a follow-up ultrasound in 4–6 weeks or sooner if indicated, referral to urology and/or nephrology, and ultrasound after birth at >48 hours to 1 month or earlier if indicated is recommended.	1.5–7.63

Short long bones (femur and humerus)	Short long bones are defined by evaluating the observed to expected ratio of bone length when compared to the biparietal diameter (BPD), not the gestational age. A fetal humerus and fetal femur with an observed to expected ratio of <90% and ≤91%, respectively, are considered short.	1.2–3.72 (femur) 2.5–5.8 (humerus)
Echogenic bowel	Increased echogenicity of the fetal bowel is defined as brightness that is similar to or greater than that of adjacent bone. Although the majority of fetuses with echogenic bowel are normal variations, it can be associated with underlying pathology, most commonly swallowed blood, aneuploidy, cystic fibrosis, growth restriction, infection (cytomegalovirus or toxoplasmosis), or a gastrointestinal malformation. Testing for chromosome abnormalities, viral infections, and carrier testing for cystic fibrosis are all appropriate evaluations. A third-trimester ultrasound (30–32 weeks) is also appropriate for monitoring fetal growth.	5.5–11.44
Increased nuchal fold ≥6 mm	This is a measurement of the tissue at the posterior fetal neck in the second trimester of pregnancy. It is considered increased when the measurement between the outer edge of the occipital bone to the outer margin of the skin measures ≥6 mm between 14–21 weeks gestation. A nuchal fold is distinctly different from a cystic hygroma or increased nuchal translucency.	11–23.30

(continued)

TABLE 5.3 Continued

Soft Marker	Description	Likelihood Ratio
Absent or hypoplastic nasal bone (NB)	The NB is seen as a bright echogenic line evaluated on a mid-sagittal view. Agenesis or hypoplasia of the NB is caused by incomplete calcification and can be seen in the first or second trimester. The size of the NB in fetuses without Down syndrome depends on gestational age (increasing in size with later gestational age). Different methods have been proposed to define nasal hypoplasia in the second trimester of pregnancy including NB measurements in the <10th or <2.5th percentile, nasal bone length (NBL) <2.5 mm or a biparietal diameter (BPD)/NBL ratio of ≥10 or ≥11. Screening performance has been shown to be better with NB measurements as a function of MoM or percentiles rather than as the BPD-to-NBL ratio. There is ethnic variability, with some populations more likely to have an absent or smaller nasal bone.	23.27–83
Ventriculomegaly, mild (10–12 mm)	Ventriculomegaly is an abnormal increased amount of cerebrospinal fluid within the ventricles of the fetal brain. It is considered abnormal when the atrial diameter of the lateral ventricles measures ≥10 mm. Between 10–12 mm is considered mild, 12–15 moderate, and >15 severe. The etiology is heterogeneous including an increased risk of aneuploidy, neural tube defects, and viral infections (cytomegalovirus and toxoplasmosis). The prognosis and management largely depend on the etiology and on the presence of associated abnormalities. A fetal MRI may be helpful.	27.52

Data from Lorente, 2017; Woodward, 2016; Bakker, 2014; Moreno-Cid, 2014; Agathokleous, 2013.

reports as low as 60% to as high as 100% (Bahado-Singh et al., 2003; Feuchtbaum et al., 2000; Yeo et al., 2003). More recent data suggests ranges closer to 90–95% (Lai et al., 2010; Sepulveda et al., 2010). Major anomalies commonly identified include congenital heart defects, brain anomalies, musculoskeletal anomalies (e.g., radial ray malformation, rocker-bottom foot, clubfoot, arthrogryposis, and clenched hands with overlapping index finger), and gastro-intestinal anomalies (e.g., omphalocele, diaphragmatic hernias). Progressive fetal growth restriction with early onset is the most common finding. Soft markers can also be identified which are al-most never in isolation, including a strawberry-shaped cavarum, choroid plexus cysts, single umbilical artery, and increased nuchal translucency or nuchal fold (Woodward et al., 2016).

Trisomy 13

Among live born infants, stillbirths, and termination in the United States, trisomy 13 has a prevalence of approximately 1 in 5,000 (Parker et al., 2010). At least 89% of pregnancies with trisomy 13 (Papp et al., 2008) will have one or more finding on an 18- to 20-week anatomy ultrasound. The hallmark finding in fetuses with tri-somy 13 is holoprosencephaly and associated facial abnormalities (cleft lip/palate, hypotelorism or cyclopia, nasal anomaly or pro-boscis), but other central nervous system abnormalities may also be identified. Other common findings include cardiac defects, enlarged echogenic kidneys, postaxial polydactyly, and fetal growth restriction. Soft markers may also be found including an increased nuchal translucency or fold, echogenic intracardiac foci, and single umbilical artery; however, these don't typically appear in isolation when the baby has trisomy 13 (Woodward et al., 2016).

Turner Syndrome

Although Turner syndrome most often results in miscarriage, it has a frequency in live births of approximately 1 in 2,500 (Stochholm et al., 2006). Fetuses with Turner syndrome may be full mono-somy X, partial monosomy X, or mosaic. Studies have shown that approximately 70% of fetuses with Turner syndrome had findings on ultrasound (Baena et al., 2004; Papp et al., 2008). Fetuses with full monosomy X showed findings approximately 90% of the time, and fetuses with mosaicism showed ultrasound anomalies only 55% of the time (Papp et al., 2008). The hallmark finding in fetuses with Turner syndrome is a cystic hygroma, with a second-trimester diagnosis more likely but a first-trimester finding also common. Other common findings include associated nonimmune hydrops, cardiac anomalies (coarctation of the aorta being the hallmark), and renal anomalies (horseshoe kidney being the hallmark). Soft markers include short femur and humerus, increased NT, and an abnormal ductus venosus flow (Woodward et al., 2016).

Triploidy

Triploidy, estimated to occur in 1–2% of all human conceptions (Jacobs et al., 1982), is a lethal chromosome abnormality that rarely results in a live birth but is common in early miscarriages. It is caused by the presence of an entire extra set of chromosomes. The extra set can be maternal (digynic) or paternal (diandric) in origin. The overall prevalence of each type varies significantly in the lit-erature, with frequency of the diandric form ranging from 20% to 85% (Joergensen et al., 2014). The different types of triploids share some common features on ultrasound (cardiac defects, syndactyly of the third and fourth digits, central nervous system anomalies, abnormal gestational sac), but also have unique presentations depending on the type. In pregnancies in which triploid is digynic, the fetuses have asymmetric growth restriction with relative mac-rocephaly and a placenta that is noncystic and either normal or small in size. In pregnancies with a dyandric triploid, the fetuses tend to have symmetrical growth restriction and placentas that are enlarged and cystic (Woodward et al., 2016). This type of placenta is often referred to as a *hydatidiform mole,* and the pregnancy as a whole may be referred to as a *partial molar pregnancy*. Early detection of triploidy and recognition of the distinction between types are important in the management of maternal health as partial molar pregnancies have been associated with maternal preeclampsia and may result in persistent trophoblastic disease, requiring follow-up (Jauniaux, 1999).

Common Ultrasound Findings

In most circumstances, a patient does not already have a known diagnosis of aneuploidy, but instead they present to genetic counseling with an ultrasound finding. See Table 5.4 for a review of some common ultrasound findings and associated risks. Table 5.5 shows the percentage risk of chromosome abnormalities with an increased NT.

Hallmark Ultrasound Findings Associated with Genetic Conditions

Many genetic conditions should be considered in the differential when a certain ultrasound finding or combination of findings is discovered. Table 5.6 lists some classic genetic conditions and their hallmark ultrasound features.

Open Neural Tube Defects

Open neural tube defects (ONTD) are a heterogeneous group of malformations occurring at a rate of 0.5–2 per 1,000 live births (Mitchell, 2005). During neurulation, the neural plate (flat sheet of cells) folds and closes to form the neural tube, the embryonic structure that develops into the brain and spinal cord. This closure is complete by the 28th day after conception or 6 weeks' gestation by last menstrual period (LMP) (Sadler, 1998). Defects arise from a failure of closure of the neural tube, resulting in conditions with a wide range of severity from lethal to surgically repairable. The

TABLE 5.4 Common ultrasound findings and risk of aneuploidy

Ultrasound Finding	Description	Risk of Aneuploidy (Most Common)
Increased nuchal translucency (NT) >95th centile	The NT is a subcutaneous fluid accumulation in the fetal neck seen between 11–14 weeks' gestation. The measurement, taken in the mid-sagittal plane with the fetal neck in a neutral position, is between the occipital bone and inner part of the fetal skin. Although an increased NT is associated with a higher risk of aneuploidy, this is a nonspecific finding that can be associated with many other genetic etiologies, congenital anomalies, and heart defects. If chromosome testing is normal, consideration of Noonan syndrome testing should be considered.	7–75%[a]
Abnormal ductus venosus flow	The ductus venosus is a vascular channel in the fetus passing through the liver and joining the umbilical vein with the inferior vena cava, which delivers blood to the right atrium of the fetal heart. It allows for oxygenated blood from the placenta to go into the fetal circulation. Doppler ultrasound is used to measure the flow of blood in this vessel. Reversal of blood flow through the ductus venosus suggests a higher risk of chromosome abnormalities and heart defects.	10× increased chance of aneuploidy – 29.6%
Choroid plexus cyst (CPC)	The choroid plexus is the part of the brain that makes cerebrospinal fluid. A choroid plexus cyst is a cyst or fluid-filled bubble inside the choroid plexus which can be likened to a blister. This is not considered a brain abnormality. It is benign, common, and often transient and may be unilateral or bilateral. A CPC is seen in 0.3–3.6% of second-trimester fetuses. Although most fetuses with an isolated CPC do not have chromosome abnormalities, 40–50% of babies with trisomy 18 have CPC.	No increased risk if isolated in a low-risk patient or if patient has low risk on screen results (T18)

Cystic hygroma	A cystic hygroma is a congenital malformation of the lymphatic system, characterized by abnormal fluid collection along the posterior neck and back of the fetus. The diagnosis is made by the presence of a cystic structure located in the occipitocervical region. Typically the size is ≥6 mm. The lesion may either be septated by internal trabeculae or not. A cystic hygroma may be identified in the first or second trimester. Chromosome abnormalities are common, but viral infections and numerous other genetic etiologies may also be the cause. Noonan syndrome testing should be offered if chromosome testing is normal, as mutations have been reported in 9–17% of cases.	50–70%[b] (45,X, T21, T18, T13)
Hydrops	Abnormal fluid accumulation in two or more fetal compartments including ascites, pleural effusion, pericardial effusion, and skin edema. May either be immune (due to red cell alloimmunization) or nonimmune (NIHF), which is seen in the majority of cases (90%). The most common etiologies of NIHF include cardiovascular causes, chromosomal anomalies, and hematologic abnormalities (e.g., alpha thalassemia). Other etiologies include fetal malformations, tumors, viral infections, placental abnormalities, and other genetic or metabolic disorders. Women with a fetus with NIHF may develop mirror syndrome (form of preeclampsia).	30–80%[c] (45X, 21, 13,18, triploidy)
Abdominal wall defect	Omphalocele and gastroschisis are abdominal wall defects that both produce herniation of the abdominal contents. An omphalocele is a membrane-covered midline defect with herniation into the base of the umbilical cord. Gastroschisis has herniation typically to the right of the umbilical cord and not covered by a membrane. Although a ruptured omphalocele is rare, this can be mistaken for gastroschisis. Differentiation between the two is important given the significant risk of chromosome abnormalities and other genetic syndromes associated with omphalocele as opposed to gastroschisis.	Minimal risk with gastroschisis, 30–40% with omphalocele (T18, T13, T21)

TABLE 5.4 Continued

Ultrasound Finding	Description	Risk of Aneuploidy (Most Common)
Holoprosencephaly (HPE)	HPE is a structural anomaly of the brain in which the developing forebrain fails to divide into two separate hemispheres and ventricles. There are three classifications of holoprosencephaly: alobar, semilobar, and lobar (listed from most to least severe). Chromosomes abnormalities are common. Other etiologies include viral infection, maternal diabetes, and maternal alcohol use. Although most cases are sporadic, X-linked, recessive, and dominant forms are described.	40–60% (T13, T18)
Cleft Lip+ or cleft palate− (CL+/−CP)	CL+/−CP are orofacial malformations. CL may be unilateral (80%) with left being more common than right. Bilateral cases and midline defects are also seen. In >80% of cases of CL, there is also a CP. Isolated CP is associated with a different genetic risks than CL+/−CP and is not often identifiable on ultrasound. Approximately 70% of CL+/−CP is isolated, and 30% have other features identified. CL+/−CP is a feature in >200 genetic syndromes.	1–6.2%[d] (T13, T18)
Atrioventricular septal defect (AVSD)	Also known as *endocardial cushion defect*. Fetuses with an AVSD have some combination of malformations of the atrial and ventricular septum, adjoining valves, and conducting system. The defect is classified as either balanced or unbalanced and partial or incomplete. Although there is a strong association with Down syndrome, other chromosomal abnormalities may also be identified.	40–70% (T21, T18, T13)

Congenital diaphragmatic hernia (CDH)	CDH is a defect in the diaphragm resulting in herniation of the abdominal contents (stomach, liver, small bowel, etc.) into the chest cavity. The defect is most commonly seen on the left side. Additional anomalies are identified in 40–50%, of which most are heart defects. Prognosis worsens if other anomalies are found, if the liver is herniated, if there is a decreased lung-to-head ratio (LHR), and if there is polyhydramnios. Chromosome abnormalities are common. Autosomal dominant, recessive, and X-linked forms have also been described.	20–25% (T18, T13, T21, tetrasomy 12p)
Duodenal atresia or stenosis	Fetal bowel obstruction that results in narrowing (stenosis) or complete blockage (atresia). Seen on ultrasound as a "double bubble." Usually seen after 20 weeks of pregnancy. Polyhydramnios develops in most but is typically not seen until after 24 weeks and is present in most by the third trimester. Associated with Down syndrome.	20–30% (T21)
Clubfoot	A general term to describe a range of anomalies resulting in a deformity of the ankle that results in a fetal foot that is fixed. Includes talipes equinovarus, talipes calcaneovalgus, and metatarsus varus (listed in order of frequency). May be unilateral or bilateral and either isolated (2/3) or complex (1/3). May be associated with other genetic conditions or open neural tube defects. Isolated cases are most likely multifactorial and the need for testing in isolated clubfoot is controversial.	1.7–30% [e] (T18, T13)

[a]See table 5 for breakdown of risk by size of nuchal translucency.

[b]Turner most common in second trimester, T21 most common in first trimester.

[c]Hydrops 30% if diagnosed at 24 weeks of gestation or later; 80% if diagnosed at 17 weeks of gestation or earlier.

[d]1.1% with CL alone and 6.2% with CL and CP were associated with chromosome abnormalities. Other anomalies almost always seen if the fetus has trisomy 18 to trisomy 13.

[e]Complex clubfoot associated with aneuploidy 10–30%, isolated clubfoot has low aneuploidy risk (1.7–2.3%).

Data from Viaris de le Sagno, 2016; Woodward, 2016; Martinez, 2010; Kagan, 2006; Mavrides, 2002; Kallen, 1996; Ota, 2016.

TABLE 5.5 Increased nuchal translucency and percentage risk of chromosome abnormality

NT (mm)	Risk of Chromosome Abnormalities	Down Syndrome	Trisomy 18	Trisomy 13	Turner Syndrome	Other Sex Chromosome Abnormalities	Triploidy	Other[a]
95th[b]–3.4	7.1	66.1	9.7	7.3	1.2	5.9	2.0	7.9
3.5–4.4	20.1	68.6	11.1	7.1	1.4	3.1	2.8	5.9
4.5–5.4	45.4	57.6	20.9	8.7	2.8	1.6	2.8	5.6
5.5–6.4	50.1	49.3	28.3	12.3	4.1	0.9	1.8	3.2
6.5–7.4	70.6	45.4	29.8	7.8	10.6	0.5	2.8	3.2
7.5–8.4	70.8	39.9	37.2	9.5	8.1	0.7	1.4	3.4
8.5–9.4	75	35.7	27.8	3.2	30.2	0.8	0.8	1.6
9.5–10.4	74.9	29.7	24.3	2.9	36.5	0	1.4	1.4
10.5–11.4	70.3	31.1	20.0	1.6	42.2	0	2.2	2.2
>11.5	70.7	14.9	12.6	0	70.1	0	0	2.3

[a]Unbalanced translocation, marker chromosomes, mosaicism, copy number variants

[b]95th centile depends on CRL

Data from Kagan, 2006.

TABLE 5.6 Hallmark Ultrasound Findings Associated with Genetic Conditions

Genetic Condition	Hallmark Feature(s)	Description
Autosomal recessive polycystic kidney disease (ARPKD)	Bilateral, enlarged, echogenic kidneys and often oligohydramnios.	An autosomal recessive condition due to mutations in the *PKHD1* gene. Prenatal diagnosis is associated with a high mortality rate, given pulmonary hypoplasia resulting from oligohydramnios. (OMIM 263200)
Beckwith-Wiedemann syndrome	Omphalocele (usually small), enlarged kidneys, macrosomia (appears large for dates), and macroglossia (protruding tongue on ultrasound).	Imprinting defect that is genetically complex. Cytogenetic (paternal duplication, translocation, inversion) in 1%, paternal UPD (~20%), methylation of IC1-maternal (~5%), loss of methylation of IC2-maternal (~55%), CDKN1C mutations (~5%). Recurrence risk depends on the cause. (OMIM 130650)
Cornelia de Lange	Severe fetal growth restriction and upper limb defects. Congenital diaphragmatic hernia is associated, but not required for diagnosis.	Genetically heterogeneous. It is an autosomal dominant condition when mutations are in the NIPBL, RED21, and SMC3 genes. Most cases are de novo (>99%) Mutations in the HDAC8 and SMC1A genes are inherited in an X-linked dominant manner and are also most likely de novo.

(continued)

TABLE 5.6 Continued

Genetic Condition	Hallmark Feature(s)	Description
L1 syndrome	Hydrocephalus in male and adducted thumbs	L1CAM gene mutations lead to a spectrum of phenotypes ranging from mild to severe. Inherited in an X-linked recessive manner. Characteristic features include hydrocephalus, intellectual disability, spasticity of the legs, and adducted thumbs. Female carriers may manifest mild features.
Meckel Gruber syndrome	Occipital encephalocele, cystic kidneys, postaxial polydactyly	An autosomal recessive condition caused by pathogenic variants in multiple genes. There is extensive clinical variability. Considered a lethal diagnosis as most babies are stillborn or die shortly after birth.
Miller Dieker	Lissencephaly	Contiguous gene deletion syndrome involving genes on chromosome 17p13.3. The size of the deletion may vary in affected individuals. Most cases are due to a sporadic deletion; however, a parental translocation may be responsible. (OMIM 247200)
Noonan syndrome	Lymphatic dysplasia (cystic hygroma or increased nuchal translucency) and polyhydramnios	Genetically heterogeneous condition inherited in an autosomal dominant manner. Most cases are due to a de novo mutation. Characterized by congenital heart disease (pulmonic stenosis and hypertrophic cardiomyopathy most common), dysmorphic facial features, webbed neck, short stature, cardiac and lymphatic abnormalities, and varying degrees of intellectual disability (most minor or normal intelligence). (OMIM 163950)

Osteogenesis imperfecta type II	Presence of multiple bone fractures. Multiple rib fractures appear as "beading." Minimal calvarial mineralization allowing brain anatomy to be "seen too well."	A group of disorders distinguished by the clinical presentations. The perinatal lethal form, type II, is autosomal dominant due to mutations in the COL1A1 and COL1A2 genes. Most of OI type II are due to de novo changes; however, gonadal mosaicism may be present in 3–5% of cases. (OMIM 166210)
Smith-Lemli-Opitz (SLO)	Early-onset fetal growth restriction, cardiac defects, underdeveloped external genitalia in males, postaxial polydactyly, and 2nd–3rd toe syndactyly	Autosomal recessive condition due to mutations in the DHCR7 gene. A severe prenatal presentation is often lethal. Survivors may have multiple medical concerns, behavioral issues, and moderate to severe intellectual disability. Low or undetectable unconjugated estriol (uE3) on maternal serum screening should prompt ultrasound looking for features. (OMIM 270400)
Thanatophoric dysplasia type I and II	Type I: curved femur often called "telephone receiver femur" and occasionally a cloverleaf-shaped skull deformity (*Kleeblattschädel*) Type II: straight femur with moderate to severe cloverleaf skull deformity (*Kleeblattschädel*)	TD is the most common lethal skeletal dysplasia with mutations in the FGFR3 gene. The vast majority of cases are due to de novo, autosomal dominant mutations. Risk of recurrence for parents who have had one affected child is not significantly increased over that of the general population; however, germline mosaicism is a theoretical possibility. (OMIM 187600, OMIM 187601)

(continued)

TABLE 5.6 Continued

Genetic Condition	Hallmark Feature(s)	Description
Tuberous sclerosis complex (TSC)	Multiple rhabdomyomas (~100% with TSC) Single rhabdomyomas (~50% with TSC)	Autosomal dominant condition caused by pathogenic variants in the TSC1 or TSC2 gene. Approximately 2/3 of cases are de novo. There is significant variability among affected individuals, which may include skin abnormalities (hypomelanotic macules, facial angiofibromas, shagreen patches, cephalic plaques, ungual fibromas); benign tumors of the brain, lungs, heart, and kidney; seizures; and intellectual disability/developmental delay. (OMIM 191100, OMIM 613254)
22q11.2 deletion	Conotruncal heart defects (tetralogy of Fallot, interrupted aortic, truncus arteriosus, ventricular septal defect).	Contiguous gene deletion syndrome involving chromosome 22q11.2. The majority are sporadic (93%). The remaining 7% are inherited in an autosomal dominant manner. Variable presentation in individuals characterized by congenital heart disease, palatal anomalies, learning disabilities, immune deficiency, hypocalcemia, and neuropsychiatric problems.

Data from Woodward, 2016; OMIM

outcomes are variable and may be difficult to predict but are loosely correlated to the size and location of the lesion. The conditions include anencephaly, craniorachischisis, iniencephaly, encephalocele, and myelomeningocele or meningocele (spina bifida).

Prenatal detection of ONTDs is largely influenced by the gestational age and type of neural tube defect. Biochemical testing by maternal serum alpha-fetoprotein (AFP) testing (Chapter 3) or amniotic fluid AFP testing with reflex to acetylcholinesterase (Chapter 4) is available. A first-trimester ultrasound has a greater than 90% chance of detecting anencephaly and approximately 80% for encephalocele, but detection of spina bifida is less likely (Taipale et al., 2003; Whitlow et al., 1999). A second-trimester ultrasound identifies virtually 100% of anencephaly. A second-trimester ultrasound also routinely evaluates for spina bifida, and examination of the entire length of the spine in the sagittal, axial, and coronal planes in combination with a cranial evaluation identifies the majority of cases: the detection rate is approximately 90–98% (Nicolaides et al., 1986). Cranial evaluation improves the detection rate as most fetuses with spina bifida have an Arnold-Chiari II malformation in which herniation of the spinal cord leads to downward displacement of the brain, resulting in obstructive ventriculomegaly, compression of the cerebellum (banana sign), and flattening of the frontal bones (lemon sign).

Approximately 2–5% of ONTDs will be syndromic due to conditions such as a chromosome abnormality (trisomy 18 or 13), and this risk is higher if other anomalies are also present (Ekin et al., 2014; Hume et al., 1986; Sepulveda et al., 2004). When not associated with a particular condition, ONTDs are thought to have a multifactorial etiology (Frey, Hauser, 2003). The genetic component is estimated at 60–70%, but few genes have yet been identified (Carter, Evans, 1973). Nongenetic risk factors include reduced folate intake, maternal anticonvulsant medication, maternal diabetes mellitus, obesity, and hyperthermia (Suarez et al., 2004). When not due to a particular syndrome, the recurrence risks for a fetus depend on the degree of relationship to the affected individual. For example, the risk of a woman having another child with an ONTD after one child is approximately 2–5%. If a woman has had two affected children, there is an estimated 10% risk to a future offspring. A fetus with a second-degree relative (aunt, uncle, half-sibling) affected has approximately a 1% risk. If the affected family member is a third-degree relative to the fetus (first cousin), the risk is estimated as 0.5%. If a parent of the fetus is affected, the risk is approximately 4% (Harper, 2011).

The risk of ONTDs can be reduced by as much as 70% with maternal supplementation of folic acid, depending on dose (Cavalli, 2008). It is recommended that women of reproductive age take 0.4 mg (400 µg) at least 1 month prior to pregnancy and throughout the first trimester. Since many pregnancies are unplanned, this folic acid supplementation should be considered regardless of intent to become pregnant, but recommended if not started previously for those contemplating pregnancy. Women who have a high risk of having a child with an ONTD because they have one themselves, have had a prior child with an ONTD, have diabetes, or are taking anticonvulsant medications are advised to take 4 mg (4,000 µg) of folic acid starting at least 1 month before conception and continuing throughout the first trimester (Toriello et al., 2011).

Of note, spina bifida occulta is a skin-covered disorder resulting from disruptions of canalization during fetal development. Canalization occurs after neural tube formation, and therefore this is a distinctly different time in development than for ONTDs. The majority of cases are asymptomatic. It is also thought to be common, affecting approximately 5–10% of the population. Because of the name, it is often confused with ONTD, which is incorrect. Spina bifida occulta does not have the same associated risks and cannot be detected prenatally by biochemical testing and rarely by ultrasound.

Teratogens

A patient may be referred to a perinatal genetic counselor to discuss an exposure to a potential teratogen during her pregnancy. "Teratogen" is the term used to describe an environmental factor or exposure that has the potential to have a harmful effect on a developing human fetus (Holmes, 2011; Nava-Ocampo, Koren, 2007).

This definition can include congenital malformations as well as other types of developmental effects such as growth restriction or functional impairment (Holmes, 2001; Običan, Scialli, 2011). These environmental factors include medications, illicit drugs, chemicals, and maternal conditions including infections (Gilbert-Barness, 2010). Although it may seem strange for a genetic counselor to address something that is mostly nongenetic, it is nevertheless a role that perinatal genetic counselors are expected to fulfill.

Teratogenic agents typically cause a distinct pattern of recognizable malformations/alterations in the fetus (Feldkamp et al., 2015). This pattern of alteration must be consistent across epidemiological studies (Buhimschi, Weiner, 2009). The effect of the teratogen should be considered "significant" and also should make biological sense (Holmes, 2011; Običan, Scialli, 2011). There must be a significant increase in the likelihood that a specific outcome will occur with the exposure when compared to the risk of an unexposed fetus (Holmes, 2010; Običan, Scialli, 2011). However, these two things are not always easy to determine. Risk can be assessed in the form of a *relative risk* or an *odds ratio*. Each specific teratogen will have a particular relative risk, which may be quite different from another teratogen's relative risk. There is currently no unanimously agreed upon minimum relative risk required to consider an agent teratogenic, though several have been proposed by the teratology community (Feldkamp et al., 2015). Additionally, an agent may be thought to be teratogenic based on observation alone, but studies may not support a biological basis for the fetal effects of the exposure. Lack of biological support may in turn not support an agent's teratogenicity (Holmes, 2011; Običan, Scialli, 2011).

To determine the teratogenicity of a particular agent, three things must be considered: dose (and route), duration, and timing (Buhimschi, Weiner, 2009; Holmes, 2011; Običan, Scialli, 2011; Polifka, 2002). *Dose* refers to the level or amount of exposure required to cause the increase in the specific outcome (Holmes, 2011; Običan, Scialli, 2011; Polifka, 2002). For most teratogenic exposures, there is a threshold level of exposure. The placenta provides a protective barrier for the fetus that any exposure must be able to cross (Buhimschi, Weiner, 2009). There is a theoretical threshold for all exposures at which an exposure below that level will cause no harmful effects while anything above that level has a direct correlation to the severity of those harmful effects (Holmes, 2011; Polifka, 2002). The route of exposure is also important as something taken orally enters the maternal bloodstream and may eventually cross the placenta whereas something applied topically does not have the same effect (Polifka, 2002).

Duration relates to the length of time the fetus was exposed to the agent (Holmes, 2010; Polifka, 2002). A one-time exposure to a teratogenic agent may have a little to no effect on a fetus while prolonged exposure to the same agent at the same dosage may increase the risk for congenital malformations (Polifka, 2002).

Last, the *timing* of the exposure must be considered. In general, there is a period during the pregnancy when the agent is most harmful to the fetus (Gilbert-Barness, 2010; Holmes, 2011; Mitchell, 2011; Običan, Scialli, 2011; Polifka, 2002). That period of time is different for each specific teratogen. In addition, different organ systems will have different periods during which they are most susceptible to exposures (Gilbert-Barness, 2010). However, in general, the period of time prior to the second week of development postconception (4 weeks by LMP) is considered the "all or none" period, the second through the ninth week is considered most important for organogenesis, and the ninth week through term (the fetal period) is important for growth and functional maturation of organ systems (Buhimschi, Weiner, 2009; Nava-Ocampo, Koren, 2007). The "all or none" period of embryonic development is termed thus because most teratogenic exposures that occur during this time period are most likely to result in a miscarriage or have no effect if the embryo survives (Buhimschi, Weiner, 2009; Nava-Ocampo, Koren, 2007; Polifka, 2002). During organogenesis, the most likely effect of a teratogenic exposure is malformation (Buhimschi, Weiner, 2009; Holmes, 2011; Nava-Ocampo, Koren, 2007; Polifka, 2002). During the fetal period of development, teratogenic exposures are more likely to cause problems with growth and maturity of an organ or system as well as with cognitive development (Buhimschi, Weiner, 2009; Holmes, 2011; Nava-Ocampo, Koren, 2007). See Figure 5.1.

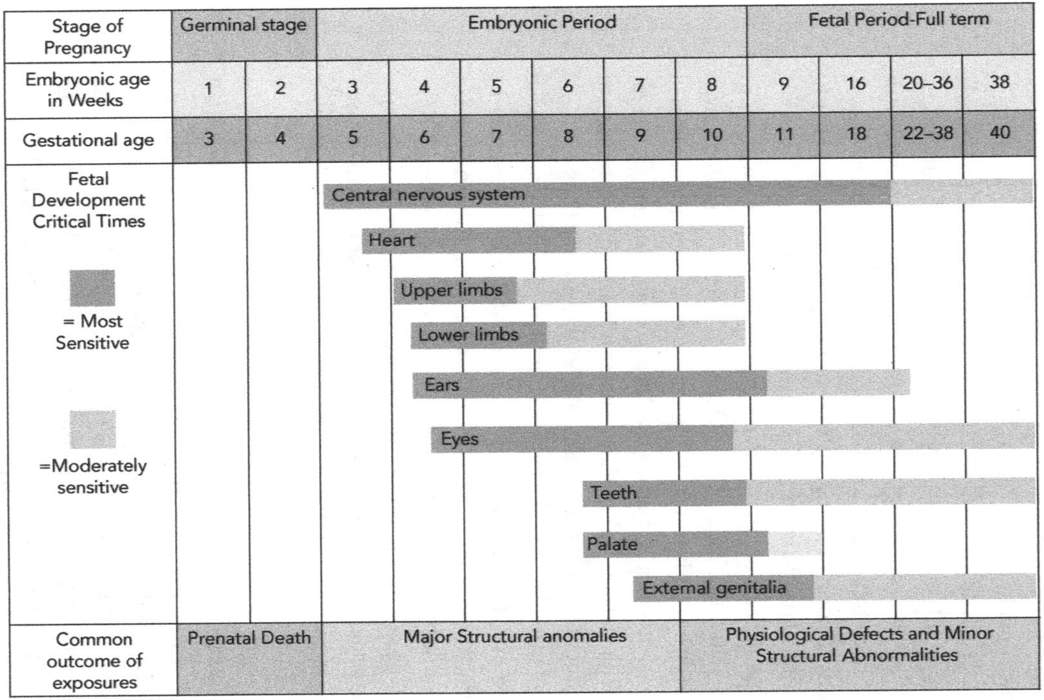

Stage of Pregnancy	Germinal stage		Embryonic Period							Fetal Period–Full term				
Embryonic age in Weeks	1	2	3	4	5	6	7	8	9	16	20-36	38		
Gestational age	3	4	5	6	7	8	9	10	11	18	22-38	40		

Fetal Development Critical Times

Central nervous system
Heart
Upper limbs
Lower limbs
Ears
Eyes
Teeth
Palate
External genitalia

= Most Sensitive

= Moderately sensitive

Common outcome of exposures: Prenatal Death | Major Structural anomalies | Physiological Defects and Minor Structural Abnormalities

FIGURE 5.1

Teratogen exposures throughout pregnancy.

From Moore, 1988

Determining the teratogenicity of an exposure can be complex. Current methodologies for determining teratogenicity are based on case-control surveillance studies and birth defects registries (Buhimschi, Weiner, 2009; Holmes, 2011; Mitchell, 2011; Rowe, 2015). Drug development companies rarely test for teratogenic effects. The truth is that most clinical trials prohibit the enrollment of pregnant or possibly pregnant participants (Buhimschi, Weiner, 2009). Instead, drugs are assumed to be likely teratogenic especially if seen to be so in animal models (Rowe, 2015). However, there are limitations in using animal models to determine teratogenicity in humans. Major malformations seen in animal models do not necessarily mean that those same malformations will occur in humans (Holmes, 2011; Nava-Ocampo, Koren, 2007). Animal models are typically given much higher doses than a human would be given in an attempt to induce malformations (Holmes, 2011). In addition, while an animal model may provide a similar biological process to that of humans, it is inevitably different and thus concrete conclusions cannot be made based on animal model data alone. These complexities are reflected in the inaccurate and often inconsistent drug classifications used by the US Food and Drug Administration (FDA) (Buhimschi, Weiner, 2009; Holmes, 2011; Rasmussen, 2012).

Counseling a patient regarding an exposure can be difficult. While it may seem that the obvious answer is to advise all women to cease taking drugs of any kind while pregnant or attempting a pregnancy, this may not always be the best solution. First, many pregnancies are unplanned and exposures may occur before a woman knows she is pregnant. Second, many women are prescribed medications for treatment of maternal illness. Recommending discontinuation will leave the illness untreated, which can have consequences. One must weigh the risks to the mother if her illness is left untreated compared to the potential risks of the exposure to the fetus, sometimes called the *motherisk approach* (ACOG, 2008; Adam et al., 2011; Mitchell, 2011; Nava-Ocampo, Koren, 2007). For example, if a woman who is taking medication to treat psychiatric illness is advised to stop taking her medication due to the potential risk to the fetus, she may become less compliant with prenatal care; expose herself to other forms of "treatment" such as herbal remedies, alcohol, or tobacco; or have difficulty bonding with the baby, as well as have an increased risk for pregnancy complications such as premature birth and low birth weight (ACOG, 2008). In addition, it would appear that some individuals may have a genetic susceptibility to a particular exposure (Holmes, 2011; Mitchell, 2011; Polifka, 2002), which may explain why some people with an exposure experience an effect and others do not. These types of genetic susceptibilities are often not able to be tested for or predicted, with only a few exceptions (Holmes, 2011). It is important to discuss all the available information with the patient, including risks and benefits of an exposure or continued exposure, to help her make the best informed decision for herself and her pregnancy (Nava-Ocampo, Koren, 2007).

Many resources are available for a genetic counselor to utilize to better guide a discussion of teratogens and exposure risks. Primary literature is always a good place to obtain the most current and up-to-date information (Holmes, 2011). However, databases and other resources are also available (Holmes, 2011; Običan, Scialli, 2011). Reprotox is an online database that can be used to view current literature summaries of nearly all pharmaceuticals and other exposures (subscription service at http://reprotox.org). MothertoBaby is another resource that can be accessed online, and it also has as an anonymous call-in system to speak with a teratogen specialist (free service at https://mothertobaby.org). Books are also available, such as *Drugs in Pregnancy and Lactation* by Briggs, Freeman, and Yaffe, although these may not be the most up-to-date resource for newer drugs on the market (Holmes, 2011). This is not a complete list of resources available, but only those that the authors have found most useful. See Table 5.7 for a list of common, known teratogenic exposures.

Recurrent Pregnancy Loss, Stillbirth, and Infertility

The American Society of Reproductive Medicine (ASRM) has proposed definitions for infertility, recurrent pregnancy loss

TABLE 5.7 Teratogen exposures

Exposure	Critical Time of Exposure	Effects
ACE inhibitors	Second and third trimesters (13 wk–term)	Neonatal respiratory distress, limb and central nervous system (CNS) defects, cardiac anomalies (patent ductus arteriosus, atrial septal defect, ventricular defect, pulmonic stenosis), calvarial hypoplasia, renal tubular dysplasia, oligohydramnios, miscarriage
Anticonvulsants/Antiepileptics (carbamazepine, valproic acid, phenytoin)	18–60 days postconception	General anticonvulsant exposure embryopathy: "cupid's bow" lip; hypertelorism; broad, depressed nasal bridge; nail hypoplasia; short nose Carbamazepine: craniofacial defects, nail hypoplasia, developmental delay Valproic acid: myelomeningocele, atrial septal defect, cleft palate, hypospadias, craniosynostosis, radial aplasia, developmental delay Phenytoin: craniofacial defects, nail and digital hypoplasia, prenatal growth deficiency, possible neuroblastomas,
Benzodiazepines	Near time of delivery	Neonatal withdrawal symptoms such as difficulty breathing and controlling body temperature, muscle weakness, irritability, sleep disturbances, tremors, jitteriness
Lithium	18–60 days postconception	Ebstein anomaly (heart defect), neonatal hypotonia, kidney and thyroid impairment
Methotrexate	6–8 weeks postconception	Meningoencephalocele, hydrocephalus, anencephaly, absent parietal bones, incomplete skull ossification, limb malformations, cleft palate
Retinoids: Oral (isotretinoin, acitretin, etretinate)	4–10 weeks postconception	Hydrocephalus, lissencephaly, severe intellectual disability, cardiac anomaly (ventricular septal defect, truncus arteriosus, double-outlet right ventricle, interrupted aortic arch, patent ductus arteriosus, tetralogy of Fallot), facial anomalies (malformed ears, cleft palate-Robin sequence, low nasal bridge, small jaw) hypotonia

Selective serotonin reuptake inhibitors (SSRIs) (Zoloft, Paxil, Lexapro, Celexa, Fluoxetine)	First trimester	General SSRI exposure: neonatal adaptation syndrome, newborn persistent pulmonary hypertension, possible heart defects Zoloft: omphalocele, atrial and ventricular septal defects Paxil: atrial and ventricular septal defects, ventricular outflow defects, anencephaly, craniosynostosis, omphalocele
	Late exposure: after 20 weeks	Neonatal mild respiratory distress, weak cry, transient tachypnea, poor tone
Thalidomide	21–40 days postconception	Limb reduction, facial hemangiomas, esophageal and duodenal atresia, cardiac anomalies (tetralogy of Fallot), renal agenesis, genital defects, facial palsy, ear anomalies, ophthalmoplegia, anophthalmia and microphthalmia, coloboma
Warfarin	6–9 weeks gestation; throughout pregnancy still a small risk	Stippled epiphyses, eye abnormalities, hypoplastic nose, distal limb hypoplasia, miscarriage/stillbirth
Maternal diabetes	Throughout pregnancy, with increased effect in the first trimester if poorly controlled	Open neural tube defects (caudal regression, anencephaly, spina bifida), heart defects (ventral septal defect, transposition of the great arteries, dextrocardia most common), defects of kidney and skeleton, VACTERL
Maternal phenylketonuria (PKU): poorly controlled	Throughout pregnancy, with increased effect in the first trimester	Intellectual disability, cardiac malformations, growth restriction, microcephaly, hip dislocation, miscarriage/stillbirth
Cytomegalovirus (CMV): primary infection	First and second trimesters, with increased effect in the first trimester	Sensorineural hearing loss, developmental delay, seizures, nonimmune hydrops, thrombocytopenia, hepatosplenomegaly, growth restriction

(continued)

TABLE 5.7 Continued

Exposure	Critical Time of Exposure	Effects
Toxoplasmosis: from cat feces and infected meat	Throughout pregnancy, though prior to 20 weeks tends to be more severe	Intellectual disability, seizures, chorioretinitis, periventricular calcifications, ventriculomegaly, hepatosplenomegaly, ascites
Rubella	<16 weeks	Sensorineural hearing loss, heart defects, cataracts, glaucoma, intellectual disability, cerebral palsy, microcephaly, growth restriction, miscarriage, stillbirth
Alcohol: fetal alcohol syndrome (FAS), typically result of alcoholic or binge drinking mothers but no amount has been found to be safe	Throughout pregnancy	FAS: intellectual disability, microcephaly, hypotonia, infant irritability, facial anomalies (thin upper vermilion of the mouth, cleft lip/palate, prominent ears), atrial septal defect General alcohol exposure: stillbirth, miscarriage, growth restriction
Nicotine/Smoking	Throughout pregnancy	Possible oral cleft, miscarriage, placental abruption, placenta previa, growth restriction, preterm delivery
Marijuana	Mostly in first trimester	Growth restriction, preterm delivery, withdrawal symptoms in neonate, nonlymphoblastic leukemia
Methylmercury: from contaminated fish	Throughout pregnancy	Brain damage (Minamata disease)

VACTERL, vertebral defects, anal atresia, cardiac defects, tracheo-esophageal fistula, renal anomalies, and limb abnormalities.

(ACOG, 1995; ACOG, 2008; Buhimschi, 2009; Gilbert-Barness, 2010; Mothertobaby.org: Obican, 2011, Polifka, 2002; Rasmussen, 2009).

(RPL), and pregnancy for the purpose of evaluation of these issues. *Infertility* is failure to achieve a pregnancy after attempting for 12 months or longer with appropriately timed intercourse or insemination (Practice Committee ASRM, 2012). RPL, also called *recurrent miscarriage*, is defined as two or more failed pregnancies (Practice Committee ASRM, 2012). In the United States, a miscarriage is defined as a pregnancy loss before 20 weeks' gestation, whereas a stillbirth is a pregnancy loss at or after 20 weeks of pregnancy (CDC, 2015). Given the possibility of incorrect information from patients who are self-reporting, a *pregnancy* is defined as one that has been confirmed by an ultrasound or histopathologic examination (Practice Committee ASRM, 2012). Pregnancy loss may be consecutive or interspersed with successful pregnancies as this does not seem to change the likelihood of identifying an underlying etiology (Laurino et al., 2005; van den Boogaard et al., 2010).

Evaluation of Pregnancy Loss and Stillbirth

Miscarriage is a common occurrence, happening in 15–25% of clinically recognized pregnancies; the incidence is greater in women of increased maternal age (ACOG no. 24; Katz, Kuller, 1994; Nybo et al., 2000). Although pregnancy loss is common, RPL only affects between 1% and 5% of couples (Practice Committee ASRM, 2012; Stirrat, 1990; van den Boogaard et al., 2010). Approximately 50% of women experiencing RPL will have an identifiable etiology to explain their history, which may include environmental and lifestyle factors, antiphospholipid syndrome, uterine abnormalities, maternal age, and hormonal or metabolic disorders (ARSM, 2012; Stephenson, 1996). Stillbirth occurs in approximately 1 in 160 pregnancies (Gregory et al., 2014). Stillbirth can also be caused by a heterogeneous list of conditions including infections, congenital anomalies, placental abnormalities, maternal medical diseases such as diabetes, and cord accidents, as well as be associated with a number of risk factors including maternal obesity, multiple gestations, poor obstetric history, and advanced maternal age

(ACOG no. 102). These etiologies are best evaluated by a perinatologist, OB provider, or reproductive endocrinologist.

Genetic factors may also contribute to a couple's history of pregnancy loss and stillbirth. The majority of first-trimester losses, approximately 60–70%, are due to sporadic chromosome abnormalities, with monosomy X, trisomy 16, trisomy 22, and triploidy being the most common (Alberman, Creasy, 1977; Choi et al., 2014; Hassold et al., 1980; Goddijn, Leschot, 2000; Pflueger, 1999). The rate of sporadic chromosome abnormalities in the products of conception (POC) of women with a history of RPL is lower, at less than 35% (Sullivan et al., 2004). The rate of chromosome abnormalities in stillbirths depends on many factors, including the presence of anatomical anomalies. Although approximately 8–13% of stillbirths will be identified with a chromosome abnormality, this rate was higher, exceeding 20%, in fetuses with growth restriction or anatomic abnormalities; in structurally normal fetuses, the risk was lower, at about 4.6% (Korteweg et al., 2008; Laury et al., 2007; Pauli et al., 1994).

Evaluation of the POC should be considered when a pregnancy loss or stillbirth occurs. Karyotyping has historically been the preferred method of testing POC. However, given a 50% cell culture failure rate where no result is obtained (Robberect, 2009), the inability of karyotype to be obtained on formalin-fixed and paraffin embedded tissue, and selective overgrowth of maternal cells leading to a normal female result (46,XX) due to culturing (Bell, 1999), microarray has been proposed as the preferred method of testing (Lomax, 2000).

Chromosome rearrangements, including Robertsonian translocations, reciprocal translocations, and pericentric or paracentric inversions, may also be responsible for a couple's history of RPL. Approximately 2–5% of couples with a history of RPL will be identified with a chromosome rearrangement (Kacprzak et al., 2016). Given this, any couple with two or more losses should be offered parental karyotype analysis to evaluate for a chromosome rearrangement (Practice Committee ASRM, 2012). If identified with a chromosome rearrangement, recurrence risk information will depend on the chromosomes involved, the size of the rearrangement, the sex of the parent who is the rearrangement carrier, and the method of ascertainment (i.e. multiple miscarriages vs. unbalanced offspring).

For those identified with a balanced reciprocal translocation, a model was developed by Dr. Carolyn Trunca at The Genetics Center to calculate the reproductive risks of miscarriage versus a live born baby. More information about this resource can be found at http://www.thegeneticscenter.com/transrsk.htm.

Evaluation of Infertility

Infertility is seen in approximately 8–15% of couples (Chandra et al., 2014; Thonneau et al., 1991). Immediate evaluation may be appropriate if physical or medical history is suggestive of a female or male infertility risk factor (Practice Committee ASRM, 2015a). If no risk factor is already known, it is appropriate to assess a couple after 12 months of attempting pregnancy when the women is younger than 35 and after 6 months if the women is 35 years of age or older. Evaluation should include a comprehensive history, physical exam, assessment of ovulatory function, structure and patency of the female reproductive tract, and a complete semen analysis to determine concentration, motility, and morphology (Practice Committee ASRM, 2012). These evaluations are best done by a reproductive endocrinologist.

Genetic counselors may also be involved in the evaluation of infertility because genetic testing may be appropriate depending on the clinical situation. However, given that "infertility" is a broad term that defines a wide range of phenotypes, the genetics and thus the testing strategies are complex and will depend on multiple factors.

Male Infertility

For a male presenting with infertility, current genetic testing options result in an etiology identified in 15–30% of cases (Walsh et al., 2009). Males presenting with nonobstructive azoospermia or severe oligozoospermia have a 10–15% and 5% risk of having a chromosome abnormality, respectively (van Assche et al., 1996). This is compared to only 1% of fertile males (Ravel et al., 2006). Klinefelter syndrome (47,XXY) accounts for the majority of cases in azoospermic males, and autosomal chromosome translocations (Robertsonian, reciprocal, inversions) are the most frequent finding in those with oligozoospermia (De Braekeleer, Dao 1991; van Assche et al., 1996). Microdeletions in regions termed the *azoospermia factors* (AZFa, AZFb, and AZFc) on the long arm of chromosome Y are also a common finding in males with infertility, seen in approximately 16% of males with either severe nonobstructive oligozoospermia or azoospermia (Foresta et al., 2001; Pryor et al., 1997). Other abnormalities commonly found include 47,XYY, 45X/46XY mosaicism, and SRY-positive 46,XX testicular disorder of sex development (Neto et al., 2016). Given the high incidence of these findings in males with nonobstructive azoospermia or severe oligozoospermia, karyotype and Y chromosome microdeletion analysis should be offered in these situations (ASRM, 2015b). If a 46,XX karyotype is identified, further testing by fluorescence in situ hybridization (FISH) analysis for the SRY gene is appropriate.

Single-gene conditions may also be responsible for male infertility. Although many conditions are possible, perhaps the most well-known is cystic fibrosis (CF) caused by mutations in the *CFTR* gene. Almost all men with CF have azoospermia due to an absence or atrophy of the vas deferens, epididymis, seminal vesicles, or ejaculatory ducts. As many as 80% of males with congenital absence of the vas deferens (CBAVD) have at least one mutation, and 50% of have two mutations in the *CFTR* gene (Yu et al., 2012). CBAVD may also be associated with renal or urinary malformations and, in these cases, is not associated with an increased risk of having CF mutations. Given this association, a male with CBAVD should have a renal sonogram and, if no renal or urinary malformation is identified, be offered testing for cystic fibrosis (Practice Committee ASRM, 2015).

Female Infertility

Women presenting with infertility may also have genetic etiologies to explain their history. Although numerous genes and syndromes have been implicated in female infertility, the most common genetic etiologies include sex chromosome abnormalities and premutation carriers of fragile-X syndrome (Rossetti et al., 2017). Turner syndrome (monosomy of the X chromosome due to partial or complete loss of one X chromosome), is the most common chromosome abnormality in women presenting with premature ovarian insufficiency (POI), but a variety of structural autosomal aberrations also may be found with relatively high frequency, including triple X (Reindollar, 2011). Given these associations, chromosome analysis and fragile-X testing may be appropriate options for testing.

Preconception Counseling

Preconception counseling is a broad term that includes identifying risk factors and providing education, counseling, and initiation of appropriate interventions prior to pregnancy. According to the ACOG, "The goal of preconception care is to reduce the risk of adverse health effects for the woman, fetus, or neonate by optimizing the woman's health and knowledge before planning and conceiving a pregnancy" (ACOG no. 313). For optimal care, the ideal time to discuss family history concerns, maternal and fetal risks associated with pregnancy, testing and management options, prevention strategies, and reproductive choices is before a pregnancy is established because it allows couples contemplating pregnancy the opportunity and time to make lifestyle or behavioral changes and to initiate a plan with their health care providers. Because every patient case is unique, the logistics, limitations, and implications can be best addressed before a pregnancy is ongoing, thus taking out the time limitation and urgency as well as allowing for accessibility to more reproductive options such as preimplantation genetic diagnosis, preimplantation genetic screening, or the use of donor gametes (egg or sperm) or having a plan in place for completing prenatal diagnosis.

Patients may come to preconception genetic counseling with either no known risk factor or they may have specific concerns (e.g., a family history of a genetic condition). A medical, pregnancy, and family history should be completed in either case to obtain all the details of the patient's situation. Other important factors to consider are the patient's desired timeline to become pregnant and how the patient intends to achieve a pregnancy (i.e., by in vitro fertilization [IVF] or naturally) as this may alter counseling and the options discussed. Maternal health conditions such as seizures, diabetes, phenylketonuria, and medication use, as well as lifestyle choices such alcohol or other substance abuse may be addressed. These concerns may need a referral for further discussion by a perinatologist, dietician, neurologist, or other health care provider. If not done previously, the couple should be encouraged to meet with their OB care provider to discuss recommendations. Routine carrier testing should be offered to all patients (see Chapter 6 for recommendations). If applicable, coordination of testing for specific conditions in the patient's personal or family history should also be arranged. Last, folic acid supplementation recommendations should be addressed.

Conclusion

Every patient a counselor works with is unique. Patients may differ in their values, decision-making styles, cultural backgrounds, personal and family history, education level, how they prefer to hear and learn information, and available support systems. Although each patient is unique, patients are referred for similar indications which were reviewed in this chapter, including age-related risks, recurrent pregnancy loss, infertility, a fetal ultrasound anomaly, teratogen exposure, or a concerning personal or family history. Patients also often want to know why they are being seen and what implications this indication has to their current or future children or pregnancies. The perinatal counselor must become expert in these indications and the implications they have for the patient in order to help the patient use the information in light of her unique needs and preferences.

References

ACOG Committee on Practice Bulletins—Obstetrics. ACOG practice bulletin: Clinical management guidelines for obstetrician-gynecologists number 92, April 2008 (replaces practice bulletin number 87, November 2007). Use of psychiatric medications during pregnancy and lactation. *Obstet Gynecol*. 2008 Apr;111(4):1001–1020.

ACOG technical bulletin. Diabetes and pregnancy. no. 200—December 1994 (replaces no. 92, May 1986). Committee on Technical Bulletins of the American College of Obstetricians and Gynecologists. *Int J Gynaecol Obstet*. 1995 Mar;48(3):331–339.

Adam MP, Polifka JE, Friedman JM. Evolving knowledge of the teratogenicity of medications in human pregnancy. *Am J Med Genet C Semin Med Genet*. 2011 Aug 15;157C(3):175–182.

Agathokleous M, Chaveeva P, Poon LC, Kosinski P, Nicolaides KH. Meta-analysis of second-trimester markers for trisomy 21. *Ultrasound Obstet Gynecol*. 2013 Mar;41(3):247–261.

Alberman ED, Creasy MR. Frequency of chromosomal abnormalities in miscarriages and perinatal deaths. *J Med Genet*. 1977 Oct;14(5):313–315.

Aylsworth AS. Genetic counseling for patients with birth defects. *Pediatr Clin North Am*. 1992 Apr;39(2):229–253.

American College of Obstetricians and Gynecologists Committee on Obstetric Practice. Committee Opinion no. 637: Marijuana use during pregnancy and lactation. *Obstet Gynecol*. 2015 Jul;126(1):234–238.

American College of Obstetricians and Gynecologists. ACOG Committee Opinion number 313, September 2005. The importance of preconception care in the continuum of women's health care. *Obstet Gynecol*. 2005 Sep;106(3):665–666.

American College of Obstetricians and Gynecologists. ACOG practice bulletin. Management of recurrent pregnancy loss. no. 24, February 2001. *Int J Gynaecol Obstet.* 2002 Aug;78(2):179–190.

American College of Obstetricians and Gynecologists. ACOG practice bulletin. Management of stillbirth. no. 102, March 2009. *Obstet Gynecol.* 2009 Mar;113(3):748–761.

American College of Obstetricians and Gynecologists and Society for Maternal-Fetal Medicine. Practice Bulletin no. 163: Screening for fetal aneuploidy. *Obstet Gynecol.* 2016 May;127(5):979–981.

Baena N, De Vigan C, Cariati E, Clementi M, Stoll C, Caballín MR, Guitart M. Turner syndrome: evaluation of prenatal diagnosis in 19 European registries. *Am J Med Genet A.* 2004 Aug 15;129A(1):16–20.

Bahado-Singh RO, Choi SJ, Oz U, Mendilcioglu I, Rowther M, Persutte W. Early second-trimester individualized estimation of trisomy 18 risk by ultrasound. *Obstet Gynecol.* 2003;101(3):463.

Bakker M, Pajkrt E, Bilardo CM. Increased nuchal translucency with normal karyotype and anomaly scan: what next? *Best Pract Res Clin Obstet Gynaecol.* 2014;28:355–366.

Barclay K, Myrskyla M. Advanced Maternal Age and Offspring Outcomes: Reproductive Aging and Counterbalancing Period Trends. *Population and Development Review.* 2016;42(1):69–94.

Basso O, Olsen J, Christensen K. Recurrence risk of congenital anomalies—the impact of paternal, social, and environmental factors: a population-based study in Denmark. *Am J Epidemiol.* 1999 Sep 15;150(6):598–604.

Baty BJ, Blackburn BL, Carey JC. Natural history of trisomy 18 and trisomy 13: I. Growth, physical assessment, medical histories, survival, and recurrence risk. *Am J Med Genet.* 1994 Jan 15;49(2):175–188.

Bell KA. Cytogenetic diagnosis of "normal 46, XX" karyotypes in spontaneous abortions frequently may be misleading. *Fertil Steril.* 1999;71:334–341.

Bennett RL, Motulsky AG, Bittles A, Hudgins L, Uhrich S, Doyle DL, Silvey K, Scott CR, Cheng E, McGillivray B, Steiner RD, Olson D. Genetic counseling and screening of consanguineous couples and their offspring: recommendations of the National Society of Genetic Counselors. *J Genet Couns.* 2002 Apr;11(2):97–119.

Berkowitz RL, Roberts J, Minkoff H. Challenging the strategy of maternal age-based prenatal genetic counseling. *JAMA*. 2006 Mar 22;295(12):1446–1448.

Bijanzadeh M. The recurrence risk of genetic complex diseases. *J Res Med Sci*. 2017 Mar 15;22:32.

Bricker L, Garcia J, Henderson J, Mugford M, Neilson J, Roberts T. Ultrasound screening in pregnancy: a systematic review of the clinical effectiveness, cost-effectiveness and women's views. *Health Technol Assess*. 2000;4:1–193.

Buhimschi CS, Weiner CP. Medications in pregnancy and lactation: part 1. Teratology. *Obstet Gynecol*. 2009 Jan;113(1):166–88.

Carter CO, Evans KA. Spina bifida and anencephalus in Greater London. *J Med Genet*. 1973;10:209–234.

Cavalli P. Prevention of neural tube defects and proper folate periconceptional supplementation. *J Prenat Med*. 2008 Oct–Dec; 2(4):40–41.

Centers for Disease Control. Fetal and perinatal mortality: United States, 2013. *Natl Vital Stat. Rep*. 2015 Jul 23;64(8).

Centers for Disease Control and Prevention (CDC). Update on overall prevalence of major birth defects-Atlanta, Georgia, 1978-2005. *MMWR Morb Mortal Wkly Rep*. 2008 Jan 11;57(1):1–5.

Cereda A, Carey JC. The trisomy 18 syndrome. *Orphanet J Rare Dis*. 2012 Oct 23;7:81.

Chandra A, Copen CE, Stephen EH. Infertility service use in the United States: data from the National Survey of Family Growth, 1982–2010. Natl Health Stat Report. 2014 Jan 22;(73):1–21.

Choi TY, Lee HM, Park WK. Spontaneous abortion and recurrent miscarriage: A comparison of cytogenetic diagnosis in 250 cases. *Obstet Gynecol Sci* 2014;57:518–525.

Crow JF. The origins, patterns and implications of human spontaneous mutation. *Nat Rev Genet*. 2000 Oct;1(1):40–47.

Crow YJ, Tolmie JL. Recurrence risks in mental retardation. *J Med Genet*. 1998 Mar;35(3):177–182.

De Braekeleer M, Dao TN. Cytogenetic studies in male infertility: a review. *Hum Reprod*. 1991 Feb;6(2):245–250.

De Souza E, Halliday J, Chan A, Bower C, Morris JK. Recurrence risks for trisomies 13, 18, and 21. *Am J Med Genet A*. 2009 Dec;149A(12):2716–2722.

Ekin A, Gezer C, Taner CE, Ozeren M, Ozer O, Koç A, Gezer NS. Chromosomal and structural anomalies in fetuses with open neural tube defects. *J Obstet Gynaecol.* 2014 Feb;34(2):156–159.

Feldkamp ML, Botto LD, Carey JC. Reflections on the etiology of structural birth defects: established teratogens and risk factors. *Birth Defects Res A Clin Mol Teratol.* 2015 Aug;103(8):652–655.

Feuchtbaum LB, Currier RJ, Lorey FW, Cunningham GC. Prenatal ultrasound findings in affected and unaffected pregnancies that are screen-positive for trisomy 18: the California experience. *Prenat Diagn.* 2000;20:293–299.

Fong KW, Toi A, Salem S, Hornberger LK, Chitayat D, Keating SJ, McAuliffe F, Johnson JA. Detection of fetal structural abnormalities with US during early pregnancy. *Radiographics.* 2004 Jan-Feb;24(1):157–174.

Foresta C, Moro E, Ferlin A. Y chromosome microdeletions and alterations of spermatogenesis. *Endocrine Rev.* 2001;22:226–239.

Frey L, Hauser WA. Epidemiology of neural tube defects. *Epilepsia.* 2003;44:4–13.

Gilbert-Barness E. Teratogenic causes of malformations. *Ann Clin Lab Sci.* 2010 Spring;40(2):99–114.

Ginsburg C, Fokstuen S, Schinzel A. The contribution of uniparental disomy to congenital development defects in children born to mothers at advanced childbearing age. *Am J Med Genet.* 2000 Dec 18;95(5):454–460.

Gregory EC, MacDorman MF, Martin JA. Trends in fetal and perinatal mortality in the United States, 2006–2012. *NCHS Data Brief.* 2014 Nov;(169):1–8.

Goddijn M, Leschot NJ. Genetic aspects of miscarriage. *Baillieres Best Pract Res Clin Obstet Gynaecol.* 2000 Oct;14(5):855–865.

Hansen JP. Older maternal age and pregnancy outcome: a review of the literature. *Obstet Gynecol Surv.* 1986 Nov;41(11):726–742.

Harper, P. *Practical genetic counseling.* 7th ed. Boca Raton, FL: Taylor and Francis; 2011:194–195.

Hassold T, Chen N, Funkhouser J. A cytogenetic study of 1000 spontaneous abortions. *Ann Hum Genet.* 1980;44:151–178.

Hassold T, Hall H, Hunt P. The origin of human aneuploidy: where we have been, where we are going. *Hum Mol Genet.* 2007 Oct 15;16 Spec no. 2:R203–R208.

Hassold T, Hunt P. To err (meiotically) is human: the genesis of human aneuploidy. *Nat Rev Genet.* 2001 Apr;2(4):280–291.

Holmes LB. Human teratogens: update 2010. *Birth Defects Res A Clin Mol Teratol*. 2011 Jan;91(1):1-7.

Hook EB. Rates of chromosome abnormalities at different maternal ages. *Obstet Gynecol*. 1981 Sep;58(3):282-285.

Hook EB, Cross PK, Schreinemachers DM. Chromosomal abnormality rates at amniocentesis and in live-born infants. *JAMA*. 1983 Apr 15;249(15):2034-2038.

Hume RF Jr, Drugan A, Reichler A, Lampinen J, Martin LS, Johnson MP, Evans MI. Aneuploidy among prenatally detected neural tube defects. *Am J Med Genet*. 1996 Jan 11;61(2):171-173.

Jacobs PA, Szulman AE, Funkhouser J, Matsuura JS, Wilson CC. Human triploidy: relationship between parental origin of the additional haploid complement and development of partial hydatidiform mole. *Ann Hum Genet*. 1982;46:223-231.

Jauniaux E. Partial moles: from postnatal to prenatal diagnosis. *Placenta*. 1999 Jul-Aug;20(5-6):379-388.

Joergensen MW, Niemann I, Rasmussen AA, Hindkjaer J, Agerholm I, Bolund L, Sunde L. Triploid pregnancies: genetic and clinical features of 158 cases. *Am J Obstet Gynecol*. 2014 Oct;211(4):370.e1-19.

Kacprzak M, Chrzanowska M, Skoczylas B, Moczulska H, Borowiec M, Sieroszewski P. Genetic causes of recurrent miscarriages. *Ginekol Pol*. 2016;87(10):722-726.

Kagan KO, Avgidou K, Molina FS, Gajewska K, Nicolaides KH. Relation between increased fetal nuchal translucency thickness and chromosomal defects. *Obstet Gynecol*. 2006 Jan;107(1):6-10.

Källén B, Harris J, Robert E. The epidemiology of orofacial clefts. Associated malformations. *J Craniofac Genet Dev Biol*. 1996 Oct-Dec;16(4):242-248.

Katz VL, Kuller JA. Recurrent miscarriage. *Am J Perinatol*. 1994 Nov;11(6):386-397. Review.

Kong A, Frigge ML, Masson G, Besenbacher S, Sulem P, Magnusson G, Gudjonsson SA, Sigurdsson A, Jonasdottir A, Jonasdottir A, Wong WS, Sigurdsson G, Walters GB, Steinberg S, Helgason H, Thorleifsson G, Gudbjartsson DF, Helgason A, Magnusson OT, Thorsteinsdottir U, Stefansson K. Rate of de novo mutations and the importance of father's age to disease risk. *Nature*. 2012 Aug 23;488(7412):471-475.

Korteweg FJ, Bouman K, Erwich JJ, Timmer A, Veeger NJ, Ravise JM. Cytogenetic analysis after evaluation of 750 fetal deaths: proposal for diagnostic workup. *Obstet Gynecol*. 2008;111:865-874.

Kotzot D. Advanced parental age in maternal uniparental disomy (UPD): implications for the mechanism of formation. *Eur J Hum Genet.* 2004 May;12(5):343–346.

Kurahashi H, Tsutsumi M, Nishiyama S, Kogo H, Inagaki H, Ohye T. Molecular basis of maternal age-related increase in oocyte aneuploidy. *Congenit Anom (Kyoto).* 2012 Mar;52(1):8–15.

Lai S, Lau WL, Leung WC, Lai FK, Chin R. Is ultrasound alone enough for prenatal screening of trisomy 18? A single centre experience in 69 cases over 10 years. *Prenat Diagn.* 2010 Nov;30(11):1094–1099.

Laurino MY, Bennett RL, Saraiya DS, Baumeister L, Doyle DL, Leppig K, Pettersen B, Resta R, Shields L, Uhrich S, Varga EA, Raskind WH. Genetic evaluation and counseling of couples with recurrent miscarriage: recommendations of the National Society of Genetic Counselors. *J Genet Couns.* 2005 Jun;14(3):165–181.

Laury A, Sanchez-Lara PA, Pepkowitz S, Graham JM Jr. A study of 534 fetal pathology cases from prenatal diagnosis referrals analyzed from 1989 through 2000. *Am J Med Genet A.* 2007;143A:3107–3120.

Lie RT, Wilcox AJ, Skjaerven R. A population-based study of the risk of recurrence of birth defects. *N Engl J Med.* 1994 Jul 7;331(1):1–4.

Lie RT, Wilcox AJ, Skjaerven R. Survival and reproduction among males with birth defects and risk of recurrence in their children. *JAMA.* 2001 Feb 14;285(6):755–760.

Liu K, Case A. Reproductive Endocrinology and Infertility Committee; Family Physicians Advisory Committee; Maternal-Fetal Medicine Committee; Executive and Council of the Society of Obstetricians. Advanced reproductive age and fertility. *J Obstet Gynaecol Can.* 2011 Nov;33(11):1165–1175.

Lomax B. Comparative genomic hybridization in combination with flow cytometry improves results of cytogenetic analysis of spontaneous abortions. *Am J Hum Genet.* 2000;66:1516–1521.

Lorente AM, Moreno-Cid M, Rodríguez MJ, Bueno G, Tenías JM, Román C, Arias Á, Pascual A. Meta-analysis of validity of echogenic intracardiac foci for calculating the risk of Down syndrome in the second trimester of pregnancy. *Taiwan J Obstet Gynecol.* 2017 Feb;56(1):16–22.

Martin JA, Kung HC, Mathews TJ, Hoyert DL, Strobino DM, Guyer B. Annual summary of vital statistics: 2006. *Pediatrics.* 2008;121(4);788–801.

Martínez JM, Comas M, Borrell A, Bennasar M, Gómez O, Puerto B, Gratacós E. Abnormal first-trimester ductus venosus blood flow: a marker of cardiac defects in fetuses with normal karyotype and nuchal translucency. *Ultrasound Obstet Gynecol.* 2010 Mar;35(3):267–272.

Maulik PK, Mascarenhas MN, Mathers CD, Dua T, Saxena S. Prevalence of intellectual disability: a meta-analysis of population-based studies. *Res Dev Disabil.* 2011 Mar–Apr;32(2):419–436.

Mavrides E, Sairam S, Hollis B, Thilaganathan B. Screening for aneuploidy in the first trimester by assessment of blood flow in the ductus venosus. *BJOG.* 2002 Sep;109(9):1015–1019.

Meyers C, Adam R, Dungan J, Prenger V. Aneuploidy in twin gestations: when is maternal age advanced? *Obstet Gynecol.* 1997 Feb;89(2):248–251.

Mitchell AA. Adverse drug reactions in utero: perspectives on teratogens and strategies for the future. *Clin Pharmacol Ther.* 2011 Jun;89(6):781–783.

Mitchell LE. Epidemiology of neural tube defects. *Am J Med Genet C Semin Med Genet.* 2005;135:88–94.

Moore KL, Persaud TVN. *Before we are born: essentials of embryology and birth defects.* Philadelphia: WB Saunders; 1998.

Moreno-Cid M, Rubio-Lorente A, Rodríguez MJ, Bueno-Pacheco G, Tenías JM, Román-Ortiz C, Arias Á. Systematic review and meta-analysis of performance of second-trimester nasal bone assessment in detection of fetuses with Down syndrome. *Ultrasound Obstet Gynecol.* 2014 Mar;43(3):247–253.

Morlando M, Bhide A, Familiari A, Khalil A, Morales-Roselló J, Papageorghiou AT, Carvalho JS. The association between prenatal atrioventricular septal defects and chromosomal abnormalities. *Eur J Obstet Gynecol Reprod Biol.* 2017 Jan;208:31–35.

Morris JK, Wald NJ, Mutton DE, Alberman E. Comparison of models of maternal age-specific risk for Down syndrome live births. *Prenat Diagn.* 2003 Mar;23(3):252–258.

Muhle R, Trentacoste SV, Rapin I. The genetics of autism. *Pediatrics.* 2004 May;113(5):e472–486.

Nava-Ocampo AA, Koren G. Human teratogens and evidence-based teratogen risk counseling: the Motherisk approach. *Clin Obstet Gynecol.* 2007 Mar;50(1):123–131.

Neto FT, Bach PV, Najari BB, Li PS, Goldstein M. Genetics of male infertility. *Curr Urol Rep.* 2016 Oct;17(10):70.

Nguyen HT, Benson CB, Bromley B, Campbell JB, Chow J, Coleman B, Cooper C, Crino J, Darge K, Herndon CD, Odibo AO, Somers MJ, Stein DR. Multidisciplinary consensus on the classification of prenatal and postnatal urinary tract dilation (UTD classification system). *J Pediatr Urol.* 2014 Dec;10(6):982–998.

Nicolaides KH, Gabbe SG, Campbell S, Guidetti R. Ultrasound screening for spina bifida: cranial and cerebellar signs. *Lancet.* 1986;328:72–74.

Nussbaum, R, McInnes, R, Huntington, W. *Thompson and Thompson Genetics in Medicine.* 7th edition. Philedelphia: Saunders Elsevier; 2007.

Nybo AA, Wohlfahrt J, Christens P, Olsen J, Melbye M. Is maternal age an independent risk factor for fetal loss? *West J Med.* 2000 Nov;173(5):331.

Običan S, Scialli AR. Teratogenic exposures. *Am J Med Genet C Semin Med Genet.* 2011 Aug 15;157C(3):150–169.

Odibo AO, Elkousy MH, Ural SH, Driscoll DA, Mennuti MT, Macones GA. Screening for aneuploidy in twin pregnancies: maternal age- and race-specific risk assessment between 9-14 weeks. *Twin Res.* 2003 Aug;6(4):251–256.

Ota S, Sahara J, Mabuchi A, Yamamoto R, Ishii K, Mitsuda N. Perinatal and one-year outcomes of non-immune hydrops fetalis by etiology and age at diagnosis. *J Obstet Gynaecol Res.* 2016 Apr;42(4):385–391.

Papp C, Szigeti Z, Tóth-Pál E, Hajdú J, Joó JG, Papp Z. Ultrasonographic findings of fetal aneuploidies in the second trimester—our experiences. *Fetal Diagn Ther.* 2008;23(2):105.

Parker SE, Mai CT, Canfield MA, Rickard R, Wang Y, Meyer RE, Anderson P, Mason CA, Collins JS, Kirby RS, Correa A. Updated national prevalence estimates for selected birth defects in the United States, 2004–2006. *Birth Defects Res Part A Clin Mol Teratol.* 2010;88:1008–1016.

Pauli RM, Reiser CA, Lebovitz RM, Kirkpatrick SJ. Wisconsin Stillbirth Service Program: I. Establishment and assessment of a community-based program for etiologic investigation of intrauterine deaths. *Am J Med Genet.* 1994;50:116–134.

Pflueger SM. Cytogenetics of spontaneous abortion. In: Gersen SL, Keagle MB, eds. *The principles of clinical cytogenetics.* Totowa, NJ: Humana Press; 1999:317–343.

Cavalli P. Prevention of Neural Tube Defects and proper folate periconceptional supplementation. *J Prenat Med.* 2008 Oct;2(4):40–41.

Polifka JE, Friedman JM. Medical genetics: 1. Clinical teratology in the age of genomics. *CMAJ.* 2002 Aug 6;167(3):265–273.

Practice Committee of American Society for Reproductive Medicine. Definitions of infertility and recurrent pregnancy loss: a committee opinion. *Fertil Steril.* 2013a Jan;99(1):63.

Practice Committee of American Society for Reproductive Medicine; Practice Committee of Society for Assisted Reproductive Technology. Recommendations for gamete and embryo donation: a committee opinion. *Fertil Steril.* 2013b Jan;99(1):47–62.

Practice Committee of the American Society for Reproductive Medicine. Evaluation and treatment of recurrent pregnancy loss: a committee opinion. *Fertil Steril.* 2012 Nov;98(5):1103–1111.

Practice Committee of the American Society for Reproductive Medicine. Diagnostic evaluation of the infertile female: a committee opinion. *Fertil Steril.* 2015a Jun;103(6):e44–50.

Practice Committee of the American Society for Reproductive Medicine. Diagnostic evaluation of the infertile male: a committee opinion. *Fertil Steril.* 2015b Mar;103(3):e18–25.

Pryor JL, Kent-First M, Muallem A, Van Bergen AH, Nolten WE, Meisner L. Microdeletions in the Y chromosome of infertile men. *N Engl J Med.* 1997;336:534–539.

Ramasamy R, Chiba K, Butler P, Lamb DJ. Male biological clock: a critical analysis of advanced paternal age. *Fertil Steril.* 2015 Jun;103(6):1402–1406.

Rasmussen SA. Human teratogens update 2011: can we ensure safety during pregnancy? *Birth Defects Res A Clin Mol Teratol.* 2012 Mar;94(3):123–128.

Rasmussen SA, Erickson JD, Reef SE, Ross DS. Teratology: from science to birth defects prevention. *Birth Defects Res A Clin Mol Teratol.* 2009 Jan;85(1):82–92.

Ravel C, Berthaut I, Bresson JL, Siffroi JP; Genetics Commission of the French Federation of CECOS. Prevalence of chromosomal abnormalities in phenotypically normal and fertile adult males: large-scale survey of over 10,000 sperm donor karyotypes. *Hum Reprod.* 2006;21:1484–1489.

Reindollar RH. Turner syndrome: contemporary thoughts and reproductive issues. *Semin Reprod Med.* 2011;29:342–352.

Robberecht C. Diagnosis of miscarriages by molecular karyotyping: benefits and pitfalls. *Genet in Med.* 2009;11(9):646–654.

Robinson WP, Langlois S, Schuffenhauer S, Horsthemke B, Michaelis RC, Christian S, Ledbetter DH, Schinzel A. Cytogenetic and age-dependent risk factors associated with uniparental disomy 15. *Prenat Diagn.* 1996 Sep;16(9):837–844.

Rossetti R, Ferrari I, Bonomi M1, Persani L. Genetics of primary ovarian insufficiency. *Clin Genet.* 2017 Feb;91(2):183–198.

Rowe T. Drugs in pregnancy. *J Obstet Gynaecol Can.* 2015 Jun;37(6):489–492.

Sachs ES, Jahoda MG, Los FJ, Pijpers L, Wladimiroff JW. Trisomy 21 mosaicism in gonads with unexpectedly high recurrence risks. *Am J Med Genet Suppl.* 1990;7:186–188.

Sadler TW. Mechanisms of neural tube closure and defects. *Ment Retard Dev Disabil Res Rev.* 1998;4:247–253.

Sepulveda W, Corral E, Ayala C, Be C, Gutierrez J, Vasquez P. Chromosomal abnormalities in fetuses with open neural tube defects: prenatal identification with ultrasound. *Ultrasound Obstet Gynecol.* 2004 Apr;23(4):352–356.

Sepulveda W, Wong AE, Dezerega V. First trimester sonographic findings in trisomy 18: a review of 53 cases. *Prenat Diagn* 2010;30:256–259.

Sharma R, Agarwal A, Rohra VK, Assidi M, Abu-Elmagd M, Turki RF. Effects of increased paternal age on sperm quality, reproductive outcome and associated epigenetic risks to offspring. *Reprod Biol Endocrinol.* 2015 Apr 19;13:35.

Snijders RJ, Sebire NJ, Nicolaides KH. Maternal age and gestational age-specific risk for chromosomal defects. *Fetal Diagn Ther.* 1995 Nov-Dec;10(6):356–367.

Snijders RJ, Sundberg K, Holzgreve W, Henry G, Nicolaides KH. Maternal age- and gestation-specific risk for trisomy 21. *Ultrasound Obstet Gynecol.* 1999 Mar;13(3):167–170.

Stephenson MD. Frequency of factors associated with habitual abortion in 197 couples. *Fertil Steril.* 1996 Jul;66(1):24–29.

Stirrat GM. Recurrent miscarriage. *Lancet.* 1990 Sep 15;336(8716):673–675.

Stochholm K, Juul S, Juel K. Prevalence, incidence, diagnostic delay, and mortality in Turner syndrome. *J Clin Endocrinol Metab.* 2006;91:3897–3902.

Stoltenberg C, Magnus P, Skrondal A, Lie RT. Consanguinity and recurrence risk of stillbirth and infant death. *Am J Public Health.* 1999a Apr;89(4):517–523.

Stoltenberg C, Magnus P, Skrondal A, Lie RT. Consanguinity and recurrence risk of birth defects: a population-based study. *Am J Med Genet*. 1999*b* Feb 19;82(5):423–428.

Suarez L, Felkner M, Hendricks K. The effect of fever, febrile illnesses, and heat exposures on the risk of neural tube defects in a Texas-Mexico border population. *Birth Defects Res Part A Clin Mol Teratol*. 2004;70:815–819.

Sullivan AE, Silver RM, LaCoursiere DY, Porter TF, Branch DW. Recurrent fetal aneuploidy and recurrent miscarriage. *Obstet Gynecol*. 2004 Oct;104(4):784–788.

Taipale P, Ammala M, Salonen R, Hiilesmaa V. Learning curve in ultrasonographic screening for selected fetal structural anomalies in early pregnancy. *Obstet Gynecol*. 2003;101(2):273–278.

Thonneau P, Marchand S, Tallec A, Ferial ML, Ducot B, Lansac J, Lopes P, Tabaste JM, Spira A. Incidence and main causes of infertility in a resident population (1,850,000) of three French regions (1988–1989). *Hum Reprod*. 1991 Jul;6(6):811–816.

Toriello HV, Meck JM; Professional Practice and Guidelines Committee. Statement on guidance for genetic counseling in advanced paternal age. *Genet Med*. 2008 Jun;10(6):457–460.

Toriello HV; Policy and Practice Guideline Committee of the American College of Medical Genetics. Policy statement on folic acid and neural tube defects. *Genet Med*. 2011 Jun;13(6):593–596.

Uehara S, Yaegashi N, Maeda T, Hoshi N, Fujimoto S, Fujimori K, *et al*. Risk of recurrence of fetal chromosomal aberrations: analysis of trisomy 21, trisomy 18, trisomy 13, and 45,X in 1,076 Japanese mothers. *J Obstet Gynaecol Res*. 1999 Dec;25(6):373–379.

van Assche E, Bonduelle M, Tournaye H, Joris H, Verheyen G, Devroey P. Cytogenetics of infertile men. *Hum Reprod*. 1996;11(Suppl 4):1–25.

van den Boogaard E, Kaandorp SP, Franssen MT, Mol BW, Leschot NJ, Wouters CH, van der Veen F, Korevaar JC, Goddijn M. Consecutive or non-consecutive recurrent miscarriage: is there any difference in carrier status? *Hum Reprod*. 2010 Jun;25(6):1411–1414.

Viaris de le Segno B, Gruchy N, Bronfen C, Dolley P, Leporrier N, Creveuil C, Benoist G. Prenatal diagnosis of clubfoot: Chromosomal abnormalities associated with fetal defects and outcome in a tertiary center. *J Clin Ultrasound*. 2016 Feb;44(2):100–105.

Walsh TJ, Pera RR, Turek PJ. The genetics of male infertility. *Semin Reprod Med*. 2009;27:124–136.

Warburton D, Dallaire L, Thangavelu M, Ross L, Levin B, Kline J. Trisomy recurrence: a reconsideration based on North American data. *Am J Hum Genet.* 2004 Sep;75(3):376–385.

Whitlow BJ, Chatzipapas IK, Lazanakis ML, Kadir RA, Economides DL. The value of sonography in early pregnancy for the detection of fetal abnormalities in an unselected population. *Br J Obstet Gynaecol.* 1999;106(9):929–936.

Whitworth M, Bricker L, Mullan C. Ultrasound for fetal assessment in early pregnancy. *Cochrane Database Syst Rev.* 2015 Jul 14;(7):CD007058.

Woodward PJ, Kennedy A, Sohaey R. *Diagnostic imaging obstetrics.* 3rd ed. Philadelphia: Elsevier; 2016:883–915.

Yeo L, Guzman ER, Day-Salvatore D, Walters C, Chavez D, Vintzileos AM. Prenatal detection of fetal trisomy 18 through abnormal sonographic features. *J Ultrasound Med.* 2003;22:581–590.

Yu J, Chen Z, Ni Y, Li Z. Cftr mutations in men with congenital bilateral absence of the vas deferens (CBAVD): a systemic review and meta-analysis. *Hum Reprod (Oxford, England).* 2012;27:25–35.

6

Carrier Screening

The purpose of carrier screening is to identify couples who are at increased risk of having children with inherited genetic conditions. Carrier screening is an important component of both preconception and prenatal care. This chapter provides information on options available, including testing based on ethnicity or targeted to the family history or clinical situation or by use of expanded carrier testing panels.

Background

Regardless of a patient's race, ethnicity, or family history, there is a risk of being a carrier of an inherited genetic condition. Carrier screening generally focuses on identifying autosomal recessive or X-linked conditions. Here, we discuss background information including who should be offered testing and when it should take place, as well as test interpretation and application of results.

Who Should Be Offered Carrier Testing?

Although specific guidelines exist on what testing should be offered to whom (see the later section "Condition-Directed or Ethnicity-Based Testing"), in general, it has been recommended that carrier testing should be offered to all women of reproductive age and their partners, if applicable (Edwards et al., 2015). Completing carrier screening when one of the biological parents is unavailable is less informative and may not be recommended, given that accurate risk assessment requires both parents. The exception is a female patient being evaluated for an X-linked condition.

Carrier Screening for Gamete Donors

All gamete (egg or sperm) donors should be screened prior to being determined eligible for donation (Edwards et al., 2015). The American Society for Reproductive Medicine (Practice Committee, 2013) has also recommended genetic screening be performed, including for cystic fibrosis (CF), on all donors, as well as other testing based on ethnicity and family history. All gamete donors should be evaluated by the current tests recommended by published guidelines at the time of the donation. Having said this, each facility has different screening practices, and many times recipients of gamete donation have to pay additional fees for donors who have completed carrier screening. Therefore, when seeing a patient who used gamete donation, carrier screening results may not be available.

Timing of Screening

Although carrier screening can be done at any time (before or during pregnancy), the ideal time to pursue carrier screening is before conception. This allows time for the option of sequential testing: first one partner is tested, and, if they screen positive for a condition, the other partner can pursue carrier testing for that condition. Sequential testing is the most cost-effective method, given that many people will not be identified as a carrier and therefore testing the patient's partner would be unnecessary in most situations. Who to test first should consider factors of family history, detection rate of the condition based on ethnicity, and if testing of X-linked conditions is being pursued. If one member of the couple is of a high-risk ethnic group, testing should begin on that individual first. For example, when the male partner is of Ashkenazi Jewish ancestry and the woman is of Caucasian ancestry, he should be screened for conditions prevalent with Ashkenazi Jewish background, and, if he is identified as a carrier, she could then be tested.

Although carrier screening prior to conception is ideal, many patients will not learn about the option of carrier screening until after they are pregnant. Depending on test turnaround time, patient's gestational age, patient preference, and if the patient is using this information for pregnancy management decisions, the sequential testing method may not be the ideal approach. Rather, concurrent testing may be more appropriate as it optimizes the time to consider diagnostic testing and reproductive options.

Evaluating Risks

During the discussion of carrier screening, many patients will want to know their risk of having an affected child. The health care provider should collect a detailed family history because there are multiple factors to consider when calculating risks, including ethnicity, personal and family history of the condition, and consanguinity, as well as what testing has already been completed. The inheritance of the condition is also a factor to consider.

Here is an example to illustrate some factors that go into this calculation:

- A couple who are both of non-Hispanic white ethnicity each has approximately a 1 in 25 carrier risk of CF without a family history (ACOG Committee on Genetics, no. 691, 2017). Given that CF is an autosomal recessive condition, if both are carriers, there is a 1 in 4 risk of having an affected child. Therefore, this couple has a 1 in 2,500 chance of an affected child (1 in 25 risk of being a carrier × 1 in 25 risk of being a carrier × 1 in 4 risk that both pass on their mutation).
- Now let's say we have a couple with the same ethnicity, but the woman reports a brother who is affected with CF: her risk is no longer 1 in 25; instead, it is 2 in 3. Without further testing, the risk of having an affected child is 1 in 150 (2/3 risk of being a

carrier × 1 in 25 risk of being a carrier × 1 in 4 risk that both pass on their mutation).

Many patients and couples have misconceptions about family history, risks, and heredity. During the conversation of risks, it is important to ask the couple about their understanding and clarify any questions or misconceptions. Perhaps one of the most common misunderstandings is thinking that one has no risk of being a carrier given an apparently negative family history. In these cases, it may be important to explain to the patient or couple that carriers often do not have any family history because these conditions can "lay hidden" in people. If they had a family history, their risk would be increased above the general population, but a negative family history does not eliminate the risk.

Another common problem is not understanding how a risk applies to each pregnancy and that the risk is random. For example, a couple with a 1 in 4 chance of having an affected child may think that this means they will have one affected child if they have four children; however, this is incorrect because *each* child has a 1 in 4 risk. Using example of gender and how some people have two girls, two boys, or one of each is often helpful to clarify how this works.

Positive Test Results

A positive test result can be frightening for patients. In these situations, if the patient is identified as a carrier of an autosomal recessive condition, consider carrier testing for her or his reproductive partner if not done previously. If a patient is identified as a carrier of an X-linked condition, further testing on her partner is not necessary to determine risks to a pregnancy. If a couple is at high risk of having a child with a condition, genetic counseling should be offered and a detailed conversation of options should be undertaken. They also should be informed that other family members are at increased risk of being carriers and that their other family members may want to pursue testing on themselves and their reproductive partners if applicable. The patients should be encouraged to share their results with their family members so appropriate testing can be pursued.

Negative Results and Residual Risks

Negative results, although seemingly simple, can be more complicated. This is because a negative result *reduces* the risk of being a carrier, but it does not eliminate it. Therefore, if testing is negative, it is not a guarantee that the patient is not a carrier or that they will have a healthy baby. The degree of risk reduction will depend on a number of factors including the detection rate, testing methodology, and ethnic background of an individual. Furthermore, carrier testing does not test for every condition possible and therefore other conditions not tested may arise.

Other Types of Results

Other types of results are also possible. Patients may be identified with a variant of uncertain significance (VUS), a variant for which it is unknown whether it represents a pathogenic mutation or a benign one. Additionally, carrier screening may identify a person who is affected with a condition. If a patient has a homozygous mutation, it can be inferred that they have the condition. Alternatively, for those with two unique mutations (compound heterozygote), further testing is needed to clarify if the mutations are *cis* (same chromosome) or *trans* (different chromosomes). Further testing of other family members may be considered, or, in some cases, condition-specific testing may be available for further clarification.

Application of a High-Risk Result

Couples or individuals who find that they are at increased risk of having a child with an inherited condition may be eligible for assisted reproductive technologies (ART) such as *in vitro* fertilization (IVF) with preimplantation genetic diagnosis (PGD). Alternatively, others may elect to use donor gametes, pursue adoption, or decide to test a pregnancy after conception by diagnostic methods (chorionic villus sampling or amniocentesis). The couple could also pursue testing on a child after birth by collection of cord blood.

Repeat Testing

Genetic testing options are evolving rapidly. Although it is ideal to test a patient for a particular condition only once, as newer and larger panels with more mutations or more conditions become available, it is possible that a patient will want to rescreen. This should be decided upon after determining if there is any added benefit to further testing.

Newborn Screening

Every state mandates testing of newborns for certain conditions in the hope of early detection and initiation of treatment. It is important to stress that carrier screening does not replace the need to have newborn screening, and newborn screening does not replace the need for carrier screening. For example, a negative newborn screen for CF on a child does not provide any information on the carrier status of the parents. Alternatively, even if parents had carrier testing for CF and both were negative, newborn screening may identify an affected infant given the possibility of the parents being carriers of less common mutations not on the testing panel completed.

Condition-Directed or Ethnicity-Based Testing

Many strategies are available to complete carrier screening. Providers must be aware of the available testing options, including offering targeted testing due to ethnicity or family history or by expanded carrier screening. Although one wants to be consistent with what is offered in a clinic, it is important to note that there are many different kinds of patients with varying desires for information; shared decision making with a patient keeping his or her personal values in mind will enable the best approach for testing. Here, we discuss current guidelines and strategies available for carrier screening. It is important, as a health care provider, to always check for updates on guidelines as they may change.

Cystic Fibrosis

CF is a common multisystem recessive condition that has variable severity characterized by a buildup of mucus leading to progressive pulmonary, gastrointestinal, and pancreatic disease, and infertility in most males due to congenital absence of the vas deferens (CBAVD). Although intelligence is unaffected, people with this condition have a shortened life span, with respiratory failure being the most common cause of death at a median survival of 37 years or 56 years in the case of a mild form of the disease (ACOG Committee on Genetics, no. 691, 2017).

The American College of Obstetricians and Gynecologists (ACOG) recommends that while carrier screening is most efficacious in the non-Hispanic white and Ashkenazi Jewish populations, testing for CF should be offered to all patients regardless of race or ethnicity (ACOG no. 691). CF screening should also be offered if there is a family history or if a prenatal ultrasound identifies a fetus with echogenic bowel, dilated bowel, or peritoneal calcifications (Langfelder-Schwind et al., 2014).

There is significant variability in the size and methodology of CF carrier screening panels available from various laboratories. In 2004, the ACOG recommended the use of a 23-mutation panel for routine carrier testing (Watson et al., 2004). The detection rate and residual risk will vary depending on ethnicity because the 23 mutations are most common in the Ashkenazi and non-Hispanic white population. Please see Table 6.1 for residual risks and detection rates based on ethnicity.

TABLE 6.1 Cystic fibrosis carrier frequency, detection rate, and residual risks

Ethnicity	CF Carrier Frequency	Detection Rate (Based on the 23-Mutation Panel) (%)	Residual Carrier Risk after a Negative Screen
Ashkenazi	1/24	94	1/380
Non-Hispanic white	1/25	88	1/200
Hispanic white	1/58	72	1/200
African-American	1/61	64	1/170
Asian-American	1/94	49	1/180

It should be noted that the R117H mutation, when identified through carrier screening, may require additional reflex testing. The R117H mutation is unique because the severity depends on which poly T variant it is inherited with. *Poly T* refers to a region of the gene that has a repeating sequence of the same genetic letter (i.e., "T"). The poly T region can either have 5T (5T repeats), 7T, or 9T. The severity of the R117H mutation is most significant if inherited with the 5T variant, less significant with the 7T, and least severe with the 9T. The ACOG recommends that, in the event that the mutation R117H is identified, a reflex test to determine the presence of a 5T should be completed.

Larger panels beyond the 23-mutation panel may be considered as they may be more appropriate for testing in individuals with ethnic backgrounds other than non-Hispanic white or Ashkenazi Jewish. Sequencing of the *CFTR* gene for routine carrier screening is not recommended but rather should be reserved for testing patients when standard carrier screening has returned negative and the patient has CF, an abnormal newborn screening, in a male with CBAVD, or having a family history when mutation documentation is unavailable. It is important to keep in mind that sequencing may reveal VUS, and therefore patients who pursue this option should be informed of this possibility.

Spinal Muscular Atrophy

Spinal muscular atrophy (SMA) is an autosomal recessive disorder characterized by progressive, proximal, and symmetrical muscle weakness and atrophy due to degeneration of motor neurons of the spine and brainstem (Crawford, Pardo, 1996). Symptoms can first appear at any time between before birth to adulthood. There is no effective treatment for the disease. SMA has been classified into five distinct subtypes (SMA 0, I, II, III, and IV) based on clinical presentation, onset of symptoms, and the maximum skill level of motor milestones achieved (Lunn, Wang, 2008; OMIM 253300). Although this classification system is useful for management and prognosis purposes, there is overlap between clinical phenotype and the molecular findings in individuals; therefore, it may be more accurate to consider this a condition with a broad spectrum. See Table 6.2 for a summary of the subtypes.

TABLE 6.2 Spinal muscular atrophy (SMA) clinical subtypes

Phenotype	Age of Onset	Life Span	Milestones Achieved
SMA 0	Prenatal	≤6 months	None
SMA I	<6 months	≤2 years, but some may live longer	Sit with support only
SMA II	6–18 months	70% alive at 25 years	Independent sitting when placed
SMA III	>18 months	Normal	Independent ambulation
SMA IV	Adulthood (20–30 years)	Normal	Normal

There are two genes associated with SMA, designted *SMN1* and *SMN2* (survival motor neuron 1 and 2, respectively). The *SMN1* and *SMN2* genes are located adjacently, on chromosome 5q13.2. There is generally one, but occasionally two, *SMN1* gene copies per chromosome. *SMN2* ranges from zero to three copies per chromosome. The *SMN1* gene is the primary disease-causing gene. Regardless of the subtype of SMA, 95% of people affected with SMA will have a homozygous deletion of exon 7 or exons 7 and 8 in the *SMN1* gene. The loss of *SMN1* function can also be due to other mechanisms such as point mutations or large deletions; therefore, the other approximately 5% may be compound heterozygotes (Hahnen et al., 1996).

The other gene, *SMN2*, acts as a modifier gene. Several studies have shown that the severity of the disease decreases with the increasing number of *SMN2* gene copies (Feldkötte et al., 2002; Prior et al., 2004; Wirth et al., 2006). However, the phenotype cannot be predicted based on *SMN2* copy number as there is overlap in clinical presentation with different *SMN2* copy numbers and clinical presentation. Having said this, most people with 0–1 copies will present with the prenatal form, 2 copies with Type I, 3 copies with type II, and 4 copies with type III.

Given that SMA has an estimated prevalence of 1 in 10,000 with a carrier frequency of 1 in 35 to 1 in 117 (see Table 6.3) depending on ethnicity (Hendrickson, 2009; Su et al., 2011; Sugarman et al., 2012) and that it occurs in all populations regardless of race or ethnicity, the American College of Medical Genetics and Genomics (ACMG) recommends offering SMA screening to everyone in the general population (Prior et al., 2008). The ACOG also recommends offering SMA carrier screening to all women who are considering pregnancy or who are currently pregnant (ACOG no. 691). Health care providers should review molecular reports of affected family members for anyone seeking carrier screening for SMA with a reported family history.

As with any test, carrier screening for SMA has limitations. Because most people with SMA will have a homozygous deletion of exon 7 or exons 7 and 8, general population carrier screening is done by a quantitative polymerase chain reaction (PCR) assay

TABLE 6.3 Spinal muscular atrophy (SMA) carrier frequency, detection rate, and residual risks

Ethnicity	Carrier Frequency	Current Detection Rate (%)	Residual Risk 2 Copies of SMN1	Residual Risk 3 Copies of SMN1
Ashkenazi Jewish ancestry	1 in 41	90	1 in 345	1 in 4,000
Asian	1 in 53	92.6	1 in 628	1 in 5,000
African-American	1 in 66	71.1	1 in 121	1 in 3,000
Hispanic	1 in 117	90.6	1 in 1,061	1 in 11,000
Caucasian	1 in 35	94.9	1 in 632	1 in 3,500

which provides *SMN1* gene dosage (McAndrew et al., 1997). This method has a detection rate of 71–94% depending on ethnicity (Hendrickson, 2009). See Figure 6.1. Carrier screening does not involve analyzing the *SMN2* copy number; however, during prenatal diagnosis this could be considered. Approximately 95% of people who are noncarriers have one *SMN1* gene on each chromosome, and therefore their dosage analysis will be two. Five percent of people who are noncarriers will have three *SMN1* genes on dosage analysis (two on one chromosome and one on the other). Of carriers, approximately 94% have one *SMN1* gene on one chromosome and none on the other and therefore this assay would identify only one *SMN1* gene. About 4% of carriers are termed "silent carriers"; they have two *SMN1* genes on one chromosome and zero on the other (McAndrew et al., 1997; Wirth et al., 1999). A silent carrier will have a dosage assay of two and appear as a noncarrier. Last, approximately 2% of carriers have a point mutation that is only detectable by sequencing (Wirth, 2000); they will also appear as a noncarrier on a gene dosage analysis. See Figure 6.1 for a summary of *SMN1* genotype configurations.

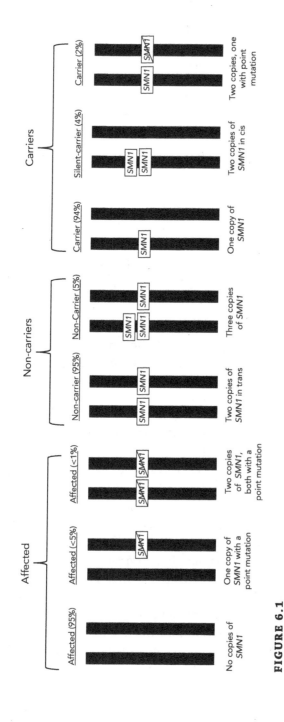

FIGURE 6.1

Spinal muscular atrophy (SMA) genotypes.

Carrier testing for parents with a prior affected child should always be done after confirming the molecular diagnosis in the child to ensure that correct testing is done. Important to note is that approximately 2% of individuals with SMA have one allele that was inherited from a carrier parent while the other was *de novo*. One should not automatically assume that a parent of a child with a homozygous deletion of exon 7 who gets two *SMN1* genes on dosage analysis is not a carrier. This child may have a *de novo* mutation or the parent may be a silent carrier.

When faced with the question of whether a person is a silent carrier or not, further testing may be necessary. Some laboratories are offering additional testing for a polymorphism in intron 7 of *SMN1*, g.27134T>G, which, if present, suggests a greater likelihood of silent carrier status (Luo et al., 2014). The polymorphism is most significant in the Ashkenazi Jewish and Asian populations but is significantly enriched in individuals in African-American, Hispanic, and Caucasian populations. Therefore, if present in the Ashkenazi Jewish or Asian population, most likely the individual is a silent carrier. However, in the African population, the risk of being a silent carrier after being identified with two *SMN1* genes and a positive polymorphism has been reported as 1 in 34; for Hispanic populations, 1 in 140; and for Caucasians, 1 in 29 (Luo et al., 2013). Further testing of other family members could also be considered for further clarification.

FMR1-Related Disorders

FMR1-related disorders are the result of alterations to the *FMR1* gene located on the X chromosome. The gene is characterized by a CGG trinucleotide repeat in the 5′ untranslated region. The number of repeats varies among individuals and is classified into four categories based on the number of the CGG repeats. Repeat lengths of 6–44 are considered normal; 45–54 repeats signify an intermediate allele, commonly called the *gray zone;* 55–200 repeats represent a premutation; and alleles with greater than 200 repeats are considered full mutations that may be either methylated or not (Fu et al., 1991). Hypermethylation of those alleles with more than 200 repeats leads to silencing of the gene (Sutcliffe et al., 1992) and an absence of fragile-X mental retardation protein (FMRP). People may also be mosaic for repeat size or methylation status of a full mutation (Pretto et al., 2014). Fewer than 1% of people with *FMR1*-related disorders have other genetic alterations, including sequence variants or large deletions of the *FMR1* gene (Suhl, Warren, 2015).

FMR1-related disorders include fragile-X syndrome, fragile-X–associated tremor ataxia syndrome (FXTAS), and *FMR1*-related premature ovarian insufficiency (POI). Fragile-X results from a full mutation. It is known to be the most common inherited form of intellectual disability and occurs in all ethnic backgrounds, affecting approximately 1 in 4,000 males and 1 in 6,000 females (ACOG no. 691). Characteristic features include moderate to severe intellectual disability in males and mild to moderate intellectual disability in females, autism spectrum disorders, macroorchidism, joint laxity, and facial features including a long face, large ears, and a prominent jaw (OMIM no. 300624). Symptoms may be milder in those who have unmethylated alleles or who are mosaic for methylation or repeat size (Pretto et al., 2014).

People with premutation or intermediate alleles are considered carriers and are not affected with fragile-X syndrome. A recent study evaluating carrier frequency for fragile-X reported that premutations were identified in 1 in 86 women with a family history of intellectual disability and 1 in 257 women with no known risk factors for fragile-X. Intermediate alleles were found in 1 in 57 women (Cronister et al., 2008).

People with intermediate alleles have no associated health consequences. Those with premutation alleles are at risk of developing FXTAS. FXTAS is characterized by late-onset, progressive cerebellar ataxia and an intention tremor. Males are more likely to have symptoms of FXTAS than are females. The estimated prevalence of FXTAS in male premutation carriers is 45.5% for men older than 50 years (Rodriguez-Revenga et al., 2009). The penetrance in women is lower, approximately 16.5% of women older than

50 years will have symptoms. (Rodriguez-Revenga et al., 2009). Female premutation carriers are also at risk of *FMR1*-related POI, which is defined as cessation of menses at less than 40 years of age, which occurs in approximately 20% of females who have an *FMR1* premutation (Wittenberger et al., 2007). The chance of identifying a premutation in a women with an isolated case of POI is 3%, and 12% for women with a personal and family history of POI (Sherman et al., 2005).

People with premutation and full mutations are at risk of having children with *FMR1*-related disorders. If a mother has a full mutation, There will be a 50% risk to each of her children to inherit the full mutation. Men who have full mutations typically do not reproduce. For premutation carriers, it is more complicated because one also has to consider the risk of a premutation to expand into a full mutation. The chance of expansion depends on the sex of the parent who has the premutation, the total number of CGG repeats, and the number of AGG interruptions. If the premutation carrier is the father, then all of his daughters and none of his sons will inherit his premutation. There may be small increases in repeat number, but they will not result in a full mutation (Ashley-Koch et al., 1998). If the mother is the premutation carrier, there is a 50% risk of passing on the abnormal allele to either a son or a daughter. There is also a risk of expansion to a full mutation, which increases as the CGG repeat size increases. The smallest allele observed to expand to a full mutation is 56 repeats (Fernandez-Carvajal et al., 2009). See Table 6.4 for a summary of the likelihood of expansion based on maternal CGG repeat size.

The stability of the allele is also influenced by the presence of AGG interruptions embedded in the CGG repeat segment (Nolin et al., 2015). In the normal population, the CGG repeats are interrupted by the AGG at positions 10 and 20. However, some people will have one or no AGG interruptions. In general, for women with a premutation with less than 90 CGG repeats, having more AGG interruptions lowers the risk of expansion to a full mutation. See Figure 6.2 for a summary of a study (Nolin et al., 2015) showing how the number of AGG repeats influenced expansion. For example,

TABLE 6.4 Risk of expansion based on maternal premutation allele size

Maternal Repeat Size	% Expansion to a Full Mutation
55–59	‹1–4
60–69	2–5
70–79	31–32
80–89	58–74
90–99	80–94
>100	94–100

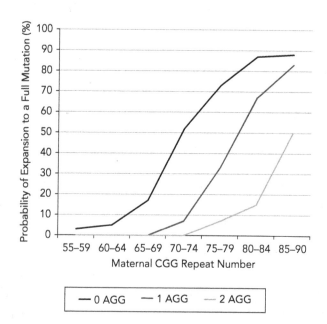

FIGURE 6.2

Stability of maternal premutation allele based on CGG repeat size and AGG interruptions.

From Nolin, 2015

a woman with 75 repeats and no AGG interruptions was shown to have a 73% chance of expansion; with 1 AGG interruption, the risk was 33%; and with 2 AGG interruptions, the risk was reduced to 7%.

Those with intermediate alleles are not at increased risk of having children with full mutations; however, the intermediate allele may be unstable and can expand into a premutation and therefore future generations may be at risk of having children with fragile-X (Nolin et al., 2011).

The ACOG (ACOG no. 691) recommends fragile-X premutation carrier screening for women with a family history of fragile-X–related disorders as well as in those with an unexplained family history of intellectual disability, developmental delay, and autism. Carrier screening should also be offered to those with either a personal or family history of unexplained POI or an elevated follicle-stimulating hormone level condition present before 40 years of age. In addition, women may request screening regardless of family history.

The gold standard for fragile-X carrier screening is PCR with Southern blot analysis. Carrier screening should be begin with PCR for the CGG repeat of the *FMR1* gene. PCR can accurately identify the CGG repeat number in the normal and lower premutation ranges, but repeat sizes larger than 100–120 may fail to be detected given PCR preferential amplification of the smaller alleles. A reflex to Southern blot can accurately determine CGG repeat sizes and has the added benefit of detecting methylation status (Basehore, Friez, 2009).

When a patient is identified as having a high risk for a child with fragile-X, she should be offered further testing. Any patient wishing to pursue prenatal diagnosis should be offered chorionic villus sampling (CVS) or amniocentesis as either sample type can yield a reliable CGG repeat number. CVS, however, has a limitation in its ability to determine methylation status accurately thus complicating interpretation and requiring a need to follow-up with amniocentesis (Willemsen et al., 2002). Therefore, any patient wishing to pursue diagnostic testing by CVS should be informed of this limitation.

Ashkenazi Jewish and French Canadian/ Cajun Ethnicity

Due to factors including genetic drift, the founder effect, and historical and social influences, people of certain ethnic backgrounds have a higher incidence of particular genetic conditions and should be offered carrier testing for those conditions. People of French Canadian or Cajun descent, as well as people of Eastern and Central European Jewish descent, termed "Ashkenazi Jewish," are at a greater risk of being carriers of Tay-Sachs disease. People with Ashkenazi Jewish ancestry are also at risk for a number of other clinically significant conditions including CF (discussed earlier), familial dysautonomia, Canavan disease, Bloom syndrome, familial hyperinsulinemia, Fanconi anemia, Gaucher disease, glycogen storage disease, Joubert syndrome, maple syrup urine disease, Niemann-Pick disease, and Usher syndrome. See Table 6.5 for a list of conditions, estimated carrier frequencies, and current guideline recommendations for those of Ashkenazi Jewish ancestry.

Importantly, carrier testing for Tay-Sachs disease can be done by molecular analysis or by hexosaminidase enzyme analysis in serum or on leukocytes. Although molecular testing has a high detection rate in those of high-risk ethnicities, for those in the general population the detection rate will be lower given the possibility of having a less common mutation not included in the testing panel. Hexosaminidase enzyme analysis has a high detection rate regardless of ethnicity. If enzyme testing is being pursued on women who are pregnant or taking oral contraceptives, it should be done on leukocytes not serum.

Hemoglobinopathies

Hemoglobinopathies are a group of disorders that affect either the structure or the production of the hemoglobin molecule. Hemoglobin is an oxygen-carrying protein found in red blood cells. It consists of four interlocking polypeptide chains, called a *tetramer*.

TABLE 6.5 Ashkenazi Jewish and French Canadian/Cajun conditions, carrier frequencies, and guidelines

Condition	Carrier Frequency Ashkenazi Jewish	Carrier Frequency in General Population	Clinical Presentation
Bloom syndrome[a,c]	1 in 100	<1 in 500	Significantly increased risk of cancer, sensitivity to sun exposure resulting in skin lesions, growth deficiency, male infertility, distinctive features and high-pitched voice (OMIM 210900)
Canavan disease[a,b]	1 in 41	<1 in 150	Severe degenerative neurological disease with symptoms appearing in the first few months of life with delayed motor milestones, hypotonia, macrocephaly, and death typically in the first decade of life (OMIM 271900)
Familial dysautonomia[a,b]	1 in 31	<1 in 500	Progressive neuronal degeneration disturbing the autonomic nervous system. This results in symptoms including pain and temperature insensitivity, vomiting crises, gastrointestinal dysfunction, frequent pneumonia, lack of tears, hypotonia, and poor regulation of blood pressure (OMIM 223900)
Familial hyperinsulinism[c]	1 in 52	<1 in 150	Too much insulin is produced by the pancreas resulting in persistent hypoglycemia resulting in seizures, hypotonia, poor feeding, and apnea; may require pancreatic resection as treatment (OMIM 256450)

(continued)

TABLE 6.5 Continued

Condition	Carrier Frequency Ashkenazi Jewish	Carrier Frequency in General Population	Clinical Presentation
Fanconi anemia C[a,c]	1 in 89	<1 in 790	This is a clinically and genetically heterogeneous condition resulting in developmental abnormalities (e.g., short stature; malformations of the eyes, ears, heart, forearms, thumbs, or kidneys), hearing loss, early-onset bone marrow failure, and a high predisposition to cancer (OMIM 227645)
Gaucher disease Type 1[a,c]	1 in 15	<1 in 100	Type 1 is the most common and presents with varying symptoms which may not be present until adulthood including hepatosplenomegaly, anemia, thrombocytopenia, lung disease, and bone abnormalities such as bone pain, fractures, and arthritis (OMIM 230800)
Glycogen storage disease type 1 A[c]	1 in 71	<1 in 150	Results in the buildup of glycogen in the liver, intestines, and kidneys. Symptoms typically manifest in the first year of life. Affected individuals may have growth delay, delayed puberty, lactic acidosis, hypoglycemia, hyperuricemia, and hyperlipidemia (OMIM 232200).
Joubert syndrome[c]	1 in 92	<1 in 500	This is a clinically and genetically heterogeneous condition. Hypoplasia of the cerebellar vermis leads to the hallmark feature of a "molar tooth" sign on magnetic resonance imaging. Features of the condition include ataxia, hypotonia, intellectual disability, and developmental delay (OMIM 213300).

Maple syrup urine disease types 1A and 1B[c]	1 in 81 (1B)	1 in 240	Metabolic disorder resulting in an inability to break down certain amino acids; the condition gets its name because the urine of affected individuals smells like maple syrup. Features include developmental delay, poor feeding, and lethargy, and, if untreated, can result in coma or death (OMIM 248600).
Mucolipidosis IV[a,c]	1 in 96	<1 in 500	Progressive neurodegenerative condition characterized by severe psychomotor delay and ophthalmologic abnormalities. People who are affected have intellectual disability and a variable life span (OMIM252650).
Niemann-Pick disease Type A[a,c]	1 in 90	<1 in 500	Severe neurological degeneration resulting in death by 3–5 years of age (OMIM 257200)
Tay-Sachs disease[a,b]	1 in 31	1 in 300 (general population; 1 in 30 French Canadian or Cajun)	Progressive neurodegenerative disease with symptoms first appearing at 3–6 months of age resulting in seizures, blindness, hearing loss, paralysis, and death by 2–3 years of age (OMIM 272800)
Usher syndrome[c]	1 in 72 and 1 in 143 (type 1F and Type 3)	Unknown	Genetically heterogeneous condition characterized by vision and sensorineural hearing loss (OMIM 302083; OMIM 276902)

[a]Recommended by the American College of Medical Genetics and Genomics (ACMG) (Gross, 2008).

[b]Recommended by the American College of Obstetricians and Gynecologists (ACOG no. 691).

[c]Conditions that should be considered by the American College of Obstetricians and Gynecologists (ACOG no. 691)

There are many different types of chains, which are termed α, β, γ, δ, ε, and ζ. The hemoglobin tetramer consists of two α chains and two non-α subunits. After the embryonic stage, there are three normal types of hemoglobin present during human life: hemoglobin A, A2, and F. Hemoglobin A has two β chains, hemoglobin A2 has two δ chains, and hemoglobin F (fetal hemoglobin) has two γ chains. Hemoglobin F is the primary hemoglobin found in a fetus. Hemoglobin F starts to decreases after 24 weeks of pregnancy, but minor amounts will be present in a healthy adult (0.8–2%). In the third trimester, hemoglobin A starts to increase and is the primary type of hemoglobin present after birth, comprising approximately 95–98%. Hemoglobin A2 is found in the adult at approximately 2–3% (Wood, 1976). Hemoglobinopathies result from mutations in the genes coding for either the β globin *(HBB)* or α globin chains *(HBA1* or *HBA2)*.

Although there are many types of structural hemoglobin variants, perhaps the most well-known is hemoglobin S (Hb S), caused by a single nucleotide change in the *HBB* gene. A person who is heterozygous has *sickle cell trait.* A person who is homozygous has *sickle cell anemia. Sickle cell disease,* however, encompasses a group of disorders characterized by the presence of at least one Hb S allele and a second abnormal allele that either affects the structure or the production of the β globin chains. For example, sickle-hemoglobin C disease (Hb SC) occurs in a person with one Hb S allele and one Hb C allele affecting the structure. Sickle β-thalassemia occurs in a person who has one Hb S allele and another for β-thalassemia which affects the production. Although symptoms are variable and may be mild or severe, characteristic features of this disorder include anemia, repeated infections, and periodic episodes of pain resulting from sickled red blood cells being stuck in blood vessels. When this happens, it results in the tissues and organs being deprived of oxygen-rich blood and can lead to permanent organ damage (Rees et al., 2010).

Thalassemias are another type of hemoglobinopathy resulting in absent or reduced production of a globin chain and are classified depending on which globin chain is affected. β-thalassemia has a reduction of β-globin production and α thalassemia has reduction in the α globin. β-thalassemia is characterized by the type of mutation or the severity of disease presentation. A mutation that causes complete absence of β-globin is noted as β°. A mutation with variable degree of reduction of globin β chain synthesis is noted as β+. People are then classified as having β-thalassemia minor, major, or intermedia. *Minor* is the term used for people who are heterozygous for a mutation (carriers). People with two mutations may be classified as having β-thalassemia major or β-thalassemia intermedia. *β-thalassemia intermedia* is clinically less severe as it results from mutations in the *HBB* gene that allow for some β-chain production, and thus some Hb A is produced. *β-thalassemia major* has a more severe clinical presentation and is due to mutations that prevent any β-globin chain production (Cao, Galanello, 2010; Olivieri, 1999).

α-Thalassemia is typically due to a common deletion of one or more of the four α globin genes, but sequence variants are also possible. There are three carrier states. The first is silent carriers who have one deletion of the α globin gene (α–/αα). The other two forms are termed *α-thalassemia trait* and can either have two deletions in *cis* (αα/– –) or trans (α–/α–). People of Southeast-Asian descent are more likely to be carriers of the *cis* form of α-thalassemia trait whereas people of African descent are more likely to have the *trans* form. There are two clinically significant states: Hb Bart syndrome is a deletion of all four α-globin genes (– –/– –), and HbH disease is a deletion of three α-globin genes (α–/– –). Hb Bart is characterized by hydrops fetalis, and most babies with this condition are stillborn or die soon after birth. Hb Bart syndrome can also lead to pregnancy complications in the mother including preeclampsia, premature delivery, and abnormal bleeding. HbH disease causes mild to moderate anemia, hepatosplenomegaly, and jaundice. The features of HbH disease usually appear in early childhood or later in life, and affected individuals typically live into adulthood (Piel, Weatherall, 2014).

Current screening recommendations are to perform a complete blood count (CBC) with red blood cell indices on all pregnant women to assess their risk of anemia and risk of a hemoglobinopathy. A hemoglobin electrophoresis should also be completed at the same time as the CBC if the patient is of a high-risk ethnicity for a hemoglobinopathy. Sickle cell disease is most common in those of African descent, with approximately 1 in 10 African Americans having sickle cell trait (Hassell, 2010). However, other high-risk ethnicities include those of Mediterranean, Middle Eastern, Hispanic, Southeast-Asian, or West Indian descent (ACOG no. 691). If a patient is identified with a low mean corpuscular volume (MCV <80 fL), and a hemoglobin electrophoresis had not been completed previously this testing should be pursued. A low MCV may also be a sign of iron deficiency anemia and therefore a serum iron ferritin level should also be evaluated in these situations. People with low MCV, normal hemoglobin electrophoresis, and normal iron studies should be evaluated for α-thalassemia by DNA-based testing as other testing cannot accurately determine α-thalassemia carriers.

Family History

Any time an individual is pursuing carrier testing of a known familial variant, records should be obtained for confirmation. Not all testing panels screen for the same conditions or the same variants in the conditions analyzed. Without confirmation of a familial mutation, the health care provider cannot guarantee that testing is being done for the correct mutation, that testing will be able to be accurately interpreted, or even that the correct condition is being tested.

A patient may also wish to pursue testing if he or she has a family member with a clinical diagnosis, but genetic testing has not been completed on that individual. Testing should ideally begin on the affected individual. Not all individuals will be identified with the genetic variant(s) that caused their condition and therefore, without confirmation in an affected family member, a negative result in a patient is difficult to interpret. The result could mean that the patient is either not a carrier, that the genetic variant is not able to be identified in the family, or that the clinical diagnosis is incorrect.

TABLE 6.6 Thalassemia genotypes, descriptions, and clinical presentation

Condition	Genotype	Description	Clinical presentation
β-thalassemia	β/β	Normal	Normal
	β°/β or β+/β	β-Thalassemia minor	Clinically asymptomatic but has minor hematologic anomalies including reduced mean corpuscular volume and elevated HbA2
	β°/β°	β-Thalassemia major	Associated with severe microcytic anemia. Symptoms appear within the first 2 years of life. Affected individuals are transfusion-dependent and may have complications of iron overload. The condition results in a s shortened life span.
	°/β+ or β+/β+	β-Thalassemia intermedia	Present at a later age, with similar but milder clinical findings. Individuals with thalassemia intermedia rarely require treatment with blood transfusion.
α-thalassemia	αα/αα	Normal	Normal
	α–/αα	α-Thalassemia silent carrier	Asymptomatic
	α–/α–	α-Thalassemia trait	Mild microcytic anemia
	αα/– –	α-Thalassemia trait	Mild microcytic anemia
	α–/– –	Hemoglobin H (HbH) disease	Moderate anemia, hepatosplenomegaly, and jaundice. Clinical features appear in early childhood. Individuals typically live into adulthood.
	– –/– –	Hemoglobin Bart hydrops fetalis (Hb Bart) syndrome	Hydrops fetalis, death in utero or shortly after birth.

A final argument about the importance of confirmation is that not all patients are accurate historians. Patients may report incorrect results and conditions, and this could lead to unnecessary or incorrect testing.

Expanded Carrier Testing

Advances in current genetic testing technologies have allowed for large numbers of conditions to be tested simultaneously, ranging from fiver to more than a hundred. Carrier screening of multiple conditions in large panels, regardless of ethnicity or family history, has been termed *expanded carrier screening* (also known as *universal carrier screening*). Although this approach to carrier testing has many advantages, it also presents unique challenges. Advantages include an increase in the amount of accessible information for patients, ability to screen when ethnicity is unknown or a person is of multiple ethnicities, ability to test for multiple conditions in the context of consanguinity, and cost-effectiveness. Disadvantages include an overwhelming amount of information and often the inclusion of conditions that are rare, have adult onset, or have little known in regards to phenotype and management.

Ethnic-specific, pan-ethnic, and expanded carrier testing are acceptable strategies for carrier testing (ACOG no. 691). A health care provider should choose an approach and be consistent within his or her practice. Guidelines have been established on the criteria for which conditions to include; that is, rather than including as many conditions as possible, expanded panels should meet census-determined criteria. Criteria that have been recommended include that the condition should have a carrier frequency of 1 in 100 or greater; have a well-defined phenotype rather than be associated with mild presentations, variable expressivity, or reduced penetrance; and should have a detrimental effect on the quality of life, cause cognitive or physical impairment, or have an onset early in life. Criteria also include recommendations to exclude adult-onset conditions; that the clinician has the ability and knowledge to calculate a residual risk when a panel is negative; and that the condition be one in which prenatal testing would be a consideration given availability of management options to improve perinatal and neonatal outcomes and to help parents prepare or make reproductive decisions (ACOG no. 691; Edwards et al., 2015; Grody et al., 2013). Expanded carrier testing does not replace the need for a CBC and hemoglobin electrophoresis when screening for hemoglobinopathies or the need for hexosaminidase A analysis for Tay-Sachs screening.

Conclusion

Offering carrier testing, including the timing of testing, identifying the best person to test, risk evaluation, and the interpretation of the results and implications for the patient, couple, pregnancy, and family is complex. Additionally, although carrier testing should be offered to all patients and gamete donors, the approach to how a health care provider offers testing may vary significantly by either offering condition- and ethnicity-based testing, expanded carrier testing, or some combination of both. Understanding available testing options as well as the implications, limitations, and benefits of each approach reviewed in this chapter can ensure that the health care provider is providing the best patient care possible.

References

ACOG Committee on Genetics. ACOG committee opinion no. 690: Carrier screening in the age of genomic medicine. *Obstet Gynecol.* 2017 March;129:e35–40.

ACOG Committee on Genetics. ACOG committee opinion no. 691: Carrier screening for genetic conditions. *Obstet Gynecol.* 2017 March;129:41–55.

Ashley-Koch AE, Robinson H, Glicksman AE, Nolin SL, Schwartz CE, Brown WT, Turner G, Sherman SL. Examination of factors associated with instability of the FMR1 CGG repeat. *Am J Hum Genet.* 1998 Sep;63(3):776–785.

Basehore MJ, Friez MJ. Molecular analysis of fragile X syndrome. *Curr Protoc Hum Genet.* 2009 Oct; chapter 9:unit 9.5.

Cao A, Galanello R. Beta-thalassemia. *Genet Med.* 2010;12:61–76.

Crawford TO, Pardo CA. The neurobiology of childhood spinal muscular atrophy. *Neurobiol Dis.* 1996;3:97–110.

Cronister A, Teicher J, Rohlfs EM, Donnenfeld A, Hallam S. Prevalence and instability of fragile X alleles: implications for offering fragile X prenatal diagnosis. *Obstet Gynecol.* 2008;111:596–601.

Edwards JG, Feldman G, Goldberg J, Gregg AR, Norton ME, Rose NC, Schneider A, Stoll K, Wapner R, Watson MS. Expanded carrier screening in reproductive medicine-points to consider: a joint statement of the American College of Medical Genetics and Genomics, American College of Obstetricians and Gynecologists, National Society of Genetic Counselors, Perinatal Quality Foundation, and Society for Maternal-Fetal Medicine. *Obstet Gynecol.* 2015 Mar;125(3):653–662.

Feldkötter M, Schwarzer V, Wirth R, Wienker TF, Wirth B. Quantitative analyses of SMN1 and SMN2 based on real-time LightCycler PCR: fast and highly reliable carrier testing and prediction of severity of spinal muscular atrophy. *Am J Hum Genet.* 2002;70:358–368.

Fernandez-Carvajal I, Lopez Posadas B, Pan R, Raske C, Hagerman PJ, Tassone F. Expansion of an FMR1 grey-zone allele to a full mutation in two generations. *J Mol Diagn.* 2009;11:306–310.

Fu YH, Kuhl DP, Pizzuti A, Pieretti M, Sutcliffe JS, Richards S. Variation of the CGG repeat at the fragile X site results in genetic instability: resolution of the Sherman paradox. *Cell.* 1991;67(6):1047–1058.

Grody WW, Thompson BH, Gregg AR, Bean LH, Monaghan KG, Schneider A, Lebo RV. ACMG position statement on prenatal/preconception expanded carrier screening. *Genet Med.* 2013 Jun;15(6):482–483.

Hahnen E, Schonling J, Rudnik-Schoneborn S, Zerres K, Wirth B. Hybrid survival motor neuron genes in patients with autosomal recessive spinal muscular atrophy: New insights into molecular mechanisms responsible for the disease. *Am J Hum Genet.* 1996;59:1057–1065.

Hassell KL. Population estimates of sickle cell disease in the US. *Am J Prev Med.* 2010 Apr;38(4 Suppl):S512–S521. doi: 10.1016/j.amepre.2009.12.022.

Hendrickson BC. Differences in SMN1 allele frequencies among ethnic groups within North America. *J Med Genet.* 2009;46:641–644.

Langfelder-Schwind E, Karczeski B, Strecker MN, Redman J, Sugarman EA, Zaleski C, Brown T, Keiles S, Powers A, Ghate S, Darrah R. Molecular testing for cystic fibrosis carrier status practice guidelines: recommendations of the National Society of Genetic Counselors. *J Genet Couns.* 2014 Feb;23(1):5–15.

Luo M, Liu L, Peter I, Zhu J, Scott SA, Zhao G, Eversley C, Kornreich R, Desnick RJ, Edelmann L. An Ashkenazi Jewish SMN1 haplotype specific to duplication alleles improves pan-ethnic carrier screening for spinal muscular atrophy. *Genet Med.* 2014 Feb;16(2):149–156.

Lunn MR, Wang CH. Spinal muscular atrophy. *Lancet.* 2008;371: 2120–2133.

Nolin SL, Brown WT, Glicksman A, Houck GE Jr, Gargano AD, Sullivan A, Biancalana V, Bröndum-Nielsen K, Hjalgrim H, Holinski-Feder E, Kooy F, Longshore J, Macpherson J, Mandel JL, Matthijs G, Rousseau F, Steinbach P, Väisänen ML, von Koskull H, Sherman SL. Expansion of the fragile X CGG repeat in females with premutation or intermediate alleles. *Am J Hum Genet.* 2003 Feb;72(2):454–464.

Nolin SL, Glicksman A, Ding X, Ersalesi N, Brown WT, Sherman SL, Dobkin C. Fragile X analysis of 1112 prenatal samples from 1991 to 2010. *Prenat Diagn.* 2011;31(10):925–931.

Nolin SL, Glicksman A, Ersalesi N, Dobkin C, Brown WT, Cao R, Blatt E, Sah S, Latham GJ, Hadd AG. Fragile X full mutation expansions are inhibited by one or more AGG interruptions in premutation carriers. Adapted from *Genet Med.* 2015 May;17(5):358–364.

Olivieri NF. The beta-thalassemias. *N Engl J Med.* 1999 Jul 8;341(2):99–109.

Pagon RA, Adam MP, Ardinger HH, Wallace SE, Amemiya A, Bean LJH, Bird TD, Ledbetter N, Mefford HC, Smith RJH, Stephens K, editors. Spinal muscular atrophy. GeneReviews® [Internet]. Seattle (WA): University of Washington, Seattle; 1993–2017. 2000 Feb 24 [updated 2016 Dec 22].

Piel FB, Weatherall DJ. The α-thalassemias. *N Engl J Med.* 2014 Nov 13;371(20):1908–1916.

Practice Committee of American Society for Reproductive Medicine; Practice Committee of Society for Assisted Reproductive Technology. Recommendations for gamete and embryo donation: a committee opinion. *Fertil Steril.* 2013 Jan;99(1):47–62.

Pretto DI, Mendoza-Morales G, Lo J, Cao R, Hadd A, Latham GJ, Durbin-Johnson B, Hagerman R, Tassone F. CGG allele size somatic mosaicism and methylation in FMR1 premutation alleles. *J Med Genet.* 2014 May;51(5):309–318.

Prior TW, Swoboda KJ, Scott HD, Hejmanowski AQ. Homozygous SMN1 deletions in unaffected family members and modification of the phenotype by SMN2. *Am J Med Genet A.* 2004;130A:307–310.

Prior TW; Professional Practice and Guidelines Committee. Carrier screening for spinal muscular atrophy. *Genet Med.* 2008 Nov;10(11):840–842.

McAndrew PE, Parsons DW, Simard LR, Rochette C, Ray PN, Mendell J, Prior TW, Burghes AH. Identification of proximal spinal muscular atrophy carriers and patients by analysis of SMNt and SMNc gene copy number. *Am J Hum Genet.* 1997;60:1411–1422

Rees DC, Williams TN, Gladwin MT. Sickle-cell disease. *Lancet.* 2010 Dec 11;376(9757):2018–2031.

Rodriguez-Revenga L, Madrigal I, Pagonabarraga J, Xunclà M, Badenas C, Kulisevsky J, Gomez B, Milà M. Penetrance of FMR1 premutation associated pathologies in fragile X syndrome families. *Eur J Hum Genet.* 2009;17:1359–1362.

Sherman S, Pletcher BA, Driscoll DA. Fragile X syndrome: diagnostic and carrier testing. *Genet Med.* 2005 Oct;7(8):584–587.

Su YN, Hung CC, Lin SY, Chen FY, Chern JPS, Tsai C, Chang TS, Yang CC, Li H, Ho HN, Lee CN. Carrier screening for spinal muscular atrophy (SMA) in 107,611 pregnant women during the period 2005–2009: a prospective population-based cohort study. *PLoS ONE.* 2011;6:e17067.

Sugarman EA, Nagan N, Zhu H, Akmaev VR, Zhou Z, Rohlfs AM, Flynn K, Hendrickson BC, Scholl T, Sirko-Osadsa DA. Allitto BA. Pan-ethnic carrier screening and prenatal diagnosis for spinal muscular atrophy: clinical laboratory analysis of >72400 specimens. *Eur J Hum Genet.* 2012;20:27–32.

Suhl JA, Warren ST. Single-nucleotide mutations in FMR1 reveal novel functions and regulatory mechanisms of the fragile X syndrome protein FMRP. *J Exp Neurosci.* 2015 Dec 8;9(Suppl 2):35–41.

Sutcliffe JS, Nelson DL, Zhang F, Pieretti M, Caskey CT, Saxe D. DNA methylation represses FMR-1 transcription in fragile X syndrome. *Hum Mol Genet.* 1992;1(6):397–400.

Watson MS, Cutting GR, Desnick RJ, Driscoll DA, Klinger K, Mennuti M, Palomaki GE, Popovich BW, Pratt VM, Rohlfs EM, Strom CM,

Richards CS, Witt DR, Grody WW. Cystic fibrosis population carrier screening: 2004 revision of American College of Medical Genetics mutation panel. *Genet Med.* 2004 Sep-Oct;6(5):387–91.

Willemsen R, Bontekoe CJ, Severijnen LA, Oostra BA. Timing of the absence of FMR1 expression in full mutation chorionic villi. *Hum Genet* 2002;110:601–605.

Wirth B, Herz M, Wetter A, Moskau S, Hahnen E, Rudnik-Schöneborn S, Wienker T, Zerres K. Quantitative analysis of survival motor neuron copies: identification of subtle SMN1 mutations in patients with spinal muscular atrophy, genotype-phenotype correlation, and implication for genetic counseling. *Am J Hum Genet.* 1999;64:1340–1356.

Wirth B. An update of the mutation spectrum of the survival motor neuron gene (SMN1) in autosomal recessive spinal muscular atrophy. *Hum Mutat.* 2000;15:228–237.

Wirth B, Brichta L, Schrank B, Lochmuller H, Blick S, Baasner A, Heller R. Mildly affected patients with spinal muscular atrophy are partially protected by an increased SMN2 copy number. *Hum Genet.* 2006;119:422–428.

Wittenberger MD, Hagerman RJ, Sherman SL, McConkie-Rosell A, Welt CK, Rebar RW. The FMR1 premutation and reproduction. *Fertil Steril.* 2007;87:456–465.

Wood WG. Haemoglobin synthesis during human fetal development. *Br Med Bull.* 1976 Sep;32(3):282–287.

7

Pregnancy Management

When a fetus is diagnosed with a genetic condition or a birth defect is detected, the pregnancy is typically recategorized as "high risk." The patient is now on a path of care that can be very different from the one she planned or envisioned for this pregnancy. The patient will have to make decisions regarding the management of the pregnancy and often in a short span of time. She will also encounter many different specialists who will help care for her and her pregnancy. While a genetic counselor may not be directly involved in every aspect of the patient's subsequent care, it is important to know the basics of what that care may include.

Reproductive Options

As with any pregnancy, there are three options available to a patient whose fetus is diagnosed with a genetic condition or congenital anomaly. These are (1) plan to give birth to and then raise the baby, who may have special needs; (2) give birth to the baby and make an adoption plan; or (3) choose to end the pregnancy (American College of Obstetricians and Gynecologists [ACOG] FAQ168). There is a fourth option in situations of congenital anomalies or a genetic diagnosis that may be lethal without intervention, which is to give birth to the baby and choose palliative care. The patient must decide which of these options is the best based on her personal values, beliefs, and goals. This decision is not usually an easy one to make, and, unfortunately, the decision often must be made in a short amount of time due to procedure, health, and legal limitations

(Bourguignon et al., 1999). The perinatal genetic counselor will work with the patient to explore these options and determine what is best for the patient, the baby, and her family.

Continuation of Pregnancy

When a patient chooses to continue the pregnancy, their obstetrical care will likely change significantly. The patient will be referred to physicians who specialize in certain areas of fetal and newborn care. The patient's obstetrician may be changed to one who specializes in high-risk pregnancies, called a *perinatologist* or *maternal–fetal medicine (MFM)* specialist. Additional imaging or fetal monitoring may be recommended. The location and plan for delivery of the baby may be changed based on the needs of the baby and mother. The patient will be advised and decisions made regarding treatment plans after the birth of the baby. Plans may also be made when the death of a baby is expected at or shortly after birth. Please see the next section for a more thorough explanation of the types of referrals that might be made.

Adoption

A patient may choose to carry the pregnancy to term but not raise the baby after delivery. It might be surprising to some that adoption is an option when a baby will likely have special needs or care requirements after birth. Many do not know that this option is available when, in fact, there are agencies that specialize in finding adoptive parents for babies with congenital anomalies, genetic conditions, and special needs. These types of agencies often work on a national scale. However, each state will have its own laws about adoption. Adoptions can be open, closed, or semi-open depending on the wishes of the biological and adoptive parents and the rules within the state and adoption agency (ACOG FAQ168). In any case, when adoption is elected, the pregnancy is managed as if the patient were electing to raise the baby after delivery. In other words, the patient's obstetric care does not differ. She will still be referred to all of the same subspecialists as a woman electing to raise the baby. Sometimes, if the adoptive parents are known prior to delivery, they may be involved in the pregnancy management and decision-making process.

Termination

Termination of a pregnancy (TOP) can have different names including *abortion, induced abortion, elective termination, therapeutic abortion*, and any combination of these. These terms are not to be confused with the term *spontaneous abortion*, which is another designation for a miscarriage. The American College of Obstetricians and Gynecologists (ACOG) uses the term *induced abortion*, which is defined as a procedure done or a medication taken to end a pregnancy (ACOG FAQS 043).

First-Trimester Termination

The specifics involved in the option of termination can vary depending on the gestational age of the fetus. First-trimester terminations can be completed either surgically or by taking medication (sometimes called a *medical termination*). Several drugs may be used alone or in combination to achieve a medical termination including prostaglandins, mifepristone (also called RU486), and methotrexate (Kulier et al., 2011). Surgical termination is performed using a procedure called *suction curettage* or *dilation and curettage (D&C)*. D&C is performed by dilation of the cervix followed by insertion of a tube into the uterus. The tube is attached to a suction or vacuum pump that is used to remove the contents of the uterus (ACOG FAQ043; Yonke, Leeman, 2013). Older techniques involved using a curette or scooping instrument to remove the contents of the uterus. After counseling, the patient is usually allowed to decide on the preferred method of termination (ACOG, 2014).

First-trimester termination, either medical or surgical, is a safe procedure (Kruse et al., 2000; Yonke, Leeman, 2013). However, as with all medical procedures, there are risks and possible side effects. Medical termination side effects commonly include heavy bleeding and severe cramping (ACOG, 2014; Kruse et al., 2000; Kulier et al., 2011). Other side effects include nausea, vomiting, diarrhea, headaches, and dizziness (ACOG, 2014; Kruse et al., 2000; Kulier et al., 2011). Risks of medical termination include the possibility of an incomplete termination and need for a subsequent surgical termination (ACOG, 2014; Kruse et al., 2000; Kulier et al., 2011). Serious risks for surgical termination, though rare, include uterine perforation, hemorrhage, or complications from anesthesia. Other risks are light bleeding, mild cramping, and infection (ACOG, 2014; Kruse et al., 2000; Yonke, Leeman, 2013).

Second-Trimester Termination

For most women whose pregnancy has been diagnosed with a genetic condition or congenital anomaly, first-trimester termination will not be an option. For these women, a second-trimester termination, which takes place after 13 weeks of pregnancy, is available. Second-trimester termination may be completed surgically or medically. A surgical termination in the second trimester is called a *dilation and evacuation (D&E)* (ACOG FAQ043). In a D&E, the cervix is prepared before the procedure, sometimes the day before. The cervix is softened and dilated using either medication, laminaria, or physical dilators. Once the cervix is dilated, the fetus is removed from the uterus by either a vacuum pump or grasping and removal using forceps and sometimes a combination of the two (ACOG, 2013; ACOG FAQ043). A suction curettage is often performed afterward to ensure that the uterus is completely empty of fetal and placental tissue (ACOG, 2013). The fetus is not typically removed completely intact using this method. If an intact fetus is desired or required for further evaluation of the fetal anatomy, then the dilation of the cervix must be larger and the procedure is usually completed over several days (ACOG, 2013). In the United States, the majority of second-trimester terminations occur by D&E (Lohr et al., 2008). Medical termination in the second trimester is similar to the technique in the first trimester, in which medications are administered to cause the uterus to contract and subsequently deliver the fetus (Wildschut et al., 2011). This technique is also called an *induction of labor*. The fetus is typically delivered intact. The provider will consider indication, effectiveness, safety, cost, patient preference, and logistics when determining the most appropriate method for termination in the second trimester (Bourguignon et al., 1999).

As with first-trimester termination, there are risks associated with each technique. Though rare, these include hemorrhage, retained products of conception (retained tissue in the uterus or incomplete termination), cervical laceration, uterine perforation or rupture, and infection (ACOG, 2013). In general, surgical termination is associated with fewer complications than medical termination in the second trimester (ACOG, 2013). Termination is not associated with reduced ability to have children in the future (Atrash, Hogue, 1990).

Later-Term Termination

Late termination is the phrase used to describe a termination of pregnancy after the second trimester, after the period of viability (the point at which the fetus has a reasonable likelihood of survival), or after the legal term limitations of the state in which the termination would take place. Many congenital anomalies and genetic conditions are not identified until much later in the pregnancy, and late termination may be the only option for some of these women (Jacobs, 2015). Late termination is not an option in all states, and special arrangements may need to be made. The procedure is very similar to a medical termination in the second trimester; however, induced demise of the fetus may be completed prior to induction and delivery with either assisted expulsion or instrumental extraction (Hern et al., 1993).

Twins

When a termination is desired in a twin gestation, the woman has the option to terminate the entire pregnancy or to terminate only the fetus with the anomaly (Ayres, Johnson, 2005). The term used for a termination in a twin pregnancy is *selective termination*, which means that one fetus in a multiple gestation pregnancy is terminated due to an anomaly or genetic diagnosis (Ayres, Johnson, 2005; Legendre et al., 2013; Yaron, 1998). This term is not to be confused with *selective reduction*, which is when a higher-order multiple gestation (two or more fetuses) is reduced to twins or a singleton early in pregnancy to reduce the risk of complications or for socioeconomic and psychological reasons (Ayres, Johnson, 2005; Legendre et al., 2013; Wimalasundra, 2010; Yaron, 1998). In a selective reduction, the fetus(es) are likely normal (Legendre et al., 2013; Yaron, 1998).

The method of selective termination is different from singleton pregnancies because the goal is to maintain the normal fetus while preventing the delivery of a live anomalous fetus (Ayres, Johnson, 2005). The method used for selective termination depends on the chorionicity of the pregnancy. In dichorionic gestations, the heart or umbilical cord of the anomalous fetus is injected with medication to stop blood circulation in that twin only while leaving the circulation of the remaining twin undisturbed (Ayres, Johnson, 2005; Legendre et al., 2013). In monochorionic gestations, the termination is completed by umbilical cord laser ablation, cord ligation, cord occlusion or transection, or an injection of a chemical into the cord of the anomalous twin to prevent blood flow to only that twin (Ayres, Johnson, 2005; Legendre et al., 2013; Wimalasundra, 2010; Yaron, 1998). It is important to note that the woman will retain the terminated fetus until delivery (Ayres, Johnson, 2005; Legendre et al., 2013). Risks associated with selective termination include loss of the entire pregnancy, preterm delivery, bleeding, and infection (Ayres, Johnson, 2005; Legendre et al., 2013; Stewart et al., 1997).

Pregnancy Management Referrals

When a patient chooses to continue her pregnancy, regardless of whether she plans to rear the baby or not, she will likely need to be seen by many subspecialists to help in the care and management of her pregnancy and in the coordination of delivery and subsequent neonatal care. Each subspecialist will bring his or her expertise into the care of the pregnancy. The collaboration of many subspecialists in the care of a high-risk pregnancy is called a *multidisciplinary approach*. Effective communication among all parties is essential in a multidisciplinary approach (Society for Maternal-Fetal Medicine (SMFM), 2014). Not all types of specialists will be utilized in all high-risk pregnancies. The organ systems involved will dictate which specialists are needed. In the next section, common types of specialists will be discussed. Depending on the indication, other subspecialists may be used who are not specifically discussed here.

The first step in this process is typically a referral to a *tertiary care center*, also called a *level IV facility* (Gagnon et al., 2009). A tertiary care center is a facility that has the capability and experience to care for the most complex and critically ill patients. In the perinatal case, a tertiary care center should be able to treat and manage the most high-risk complications of pregnancy (ACOG/SMFM, 2015). This may include a complete transfer of obstetric care and location of delivery or simply a consultation with the subspecialist to assist the patient and her regular obstetric provider in the management of her pregnancy.

Maternal–Fetal Medicine Specialist

A MFM specialist, also called a perinatologist, is an obstetrician-gynecologist who has special training and expertise in the diagnosis and treatment of women who have complications of pregnancy, including fetal issues or maternal conditions (Society for Maternal-Fetal Medicine (SMFM), 2014). An MFM will provide consultations, co-management, or direct care for women with complicated pregnancies. A consultation usually consists of a single visit with the MFM, when he or she will make recommendations to the patient and her primary OB for care and/or subsequent evaluations based on the indication. Co-management with a primary OB and an MFM is when the two physicians work together to care for and manage the pregnancy. In this situation, the patient's primary OB will be responsible for regular obstetric care and delivery, while the MFM will be responsible for the care of the condition or complication, including testing and additional evaluations. When a complete transfer of care occurs, the MFM becomes the patient's primary obstetrician. The MFM will coordinate all of the patient's care, including making appropriate referrals to other subspecialties, ordering maternal or fetal testing, performing the delivery, and providing postpartum care of the woman (Society for Maternal-Fetal Medicine (SMFM), 2014). Genetic counselors usually work very closely with the MFM to assist with testing and support.

Specialized Imaging

For most pregnancies, traditional ultrasound, or 2D ultrasound, is an adequate method for assessing the fetus. When a congenital anomaly is found or suspected, other imaging modalities may offer a more high-definition image for a better assessment.

3D Ultrasound

A 3D ultrasound is basically an expansion of the 2D ultrasound. By using a specialized transducer, two-dimensional images, similar to those obtained by a traditional ultrasound, are manipulated by a software program to create three-dimensional images. This is done by volume data acquisition as opposed to pixel data used in the 2D method. These 3D images are complementary to the 2D ultrasound and can be particularly useful in the assessment of fetal face and limbs when an anomaly is suspected. 3D ultrasound does not replace the use of a 2D ultrasound (Sepulveda et al., 2012).

Echocardiography

A fetal echocardiogram is a specific type of ultrasound that is designed to provide anatomical detail of the fetal cardiovascular system beyond that of the standard 2D obstetrical ultrasound (Rychick et al., 2004). The fetal echocardiogram, sometimes called a *fetal echo*, is used to either identify or confirm a congenital heart defect as well as to characterize it (Rogers et al., 2013). The fetal echo uses sound waves and the echo of those sound waves as they bounce off the fetal heart to create a dynamic image of the heart. Interpretation of this image requires specialized skill and knowledge of the fetal cardiovascular system (Rychick et al., 2004). The fetal echo has the ability to provide Doppler imaging as well, which allows for the assessment of movement and flow of blood throughout the fetal cardiovascular system (Rychick et al., 2004). A fetal echocardiogram is best performed between 18 and 22 weeks of gestation (Rychick et al., 2004).

Magnetic Resonance Imaging

As briefly mentioned in Chapter 1, the fetal magnetic resonance imaging (MRI) is another imaging modality. MRI generates high-quality images by using electromagnetic pulses to measure the properties of hydrogen atoms found in a targeted body tissue. A magnetic field is generated followed by a radiofrequency pulse. The tissue releases a detectable electromagnetic pulse that is measurable by a computer. Different tissues have varying hydrogen content and release electromagnetic energy at different levels. The computer measures the intensity of the electromagnetic response of the tissue and then generates a representative image of that region (Sepulveda et al., 2012). The result will be a highly detailed image of the fetal anatomy. Common indications for a fetal MRI include central nervous system anomalies, diaphragmatic hernia, myelomeningocele, neck and face masses, possible airway obstruction, lung masses or sequestration, gastrointestinal anomalies, and genitourinary anomalies (Glenn, Coakley, 2009; Wright et al., 2010). MRI also has the benefit of being able to obtain images of the fetus when oligohydramnios is present and 2D ultrasound would be limited (Wright et al., 2010).

Cardiology

A referral to pediatric cardiology is made when a fetus has a congenital heart defect (CHD). As identification and management of CHD has been shown to have a positive impact on the outcome of newborns, the pediatric cardiologist plays a crucial role in the management of these pregnancies (Sanapo et al., 2016). Assessment of the fetal heart may include several fetal echocardiograms to evaluate for possible changes in the CHD (Sanapo et al., 2016). The cardiologist will provide the patient with detailed information regarding the type of CHD the fetus has, as well as the prognosis. They may make recommendations for the location, timing, and mode of delivery of the baby, often including delivery at a tertiary care facility (Sanapo et al., 2016). The cardiology team will also provide information and recommendations for treatment and/or surgery after birth, if needed.

Neonatology

A neonatologist is a pediatric specialist who manages the care of a high-risk infant after delivery (Davis et al., 2014). Like the MFM, the neonatologist will obtain information from many other subspecialists to formulate a comprehensive plan for the care and treatment of a high-risk newborn as a complete picture. The goal of the neonatologist is to coordinate the continuation of care from fetus to neonate. This includes predelivery guidance for the parents, such as prognosis after birth; delivery room processes; possible hospitalization of the newborn after delivery; methods for diagnosis, surveillance, and monitoring; transition to home; and follow-up care. The concept of palliative or comfort care may be addressed by the neonatologist in situations where prognosis is poor (Davis et al., 2014).

Fetal Surgery or Intervention

Fetal surgery is a surgical intervention completed while the fetus is still *in utero* (in the uterus) to repair certain birth defects instead of undertaking such repair after birth. The decision to perform fetal surgery includes considerations for both mother and fetus (Sudhakaran et al., 2012). In *open fetal surgeries*, the uterus is opened up with an incision through the maternal abdomen to reach the fetus. *Closed fetal surgeries*, which are less invasive, require a smaller incision in the uterus to reach the fetus and are guided by a scope (called a fetoscope) and ultrasound (Sudhakaran et al., 2012; Wenstrom, Carr, 2014). A common open fetal surgery is for spina bifida (myelomeningocele) (Adzick et al., 2011; Peranteau, Adzick, 2016). Fetoscopic surgical indications include twin–twin transfusion syndrome (TTTS), twin reversed arterial perfusion sequence (TRAP sequence), urinary tract obstruction, and fetal tumors (Sudhakaran et al., 2012; Wenstrom, Carr, 2014). Other congenital anomalies may also be amenable to fetal interventions.

Pediatric Surgery

A pediatric surgeon specializes in operating on infants and children, typically ranging from newborns to teenagers (Colombani, 2003). Pediatric surgeons will manage the pre- and postoperative care of those born with a range of congenital abnormalities including but not limited to abdominal wall defects, diaphragmatic hernia, and open neural tube defects (American Academy of Pediatrics healthychildren.org, 2015). Preoperative care can include discussions with the family and the MFM prior to the birth of the baby. Discussions will include likely surgical outcome, possible complications, subsequent management, and follow-up (Benachi, Sarnacki, 2014).

Pediatric Specialists

As with adult medical care, there are subspecialists in pediatric health care. Children often have specific and unique treatment needs when compared to adults, and there are many subspecialties within pediatric care. The type of subspecialist that a pregnant woman may meet with depends on the organ system that is or may be affected by the genetic condition or congenital anomaly present in the fetus. Many of these subspecialties will overlap with pediatric surgery. For example, a pediatric urologist will treat an infant with an anomaly involving the genitals or the urinary tract (kidney, ureter, and bladder). A pediatric neurologist will treat an infant with problems involving the nervous system, such as hydrocephalus and muscular dystrophy. A pediatric orthopedic surgeon will treat infants with musculoskeletal conditions including clubfoot and limb abnormalities. A pediatric geneticist will diagnose, treat, and manage children with all types of genetic conditions including Down syndrome, achondroplasia, and fragile-X syndrome (American Academy of Pediatrics healthychildren.org, 2015).

Pathology and Autopsy

When a fetus dies in utero (intrauterine fetal demise), is stillborn, dies shortly after birth, or a termination is elected, an autopsy is often performed to determine the cause of death, identify and characterize congenital structural abnormalities, provide or refute a diagnosis and possible recurrence risk, and help in the management of future pregnancies (Désilets et al., 2011; Dickinson et al., 2011; Miller et al., 2016). A pathologist is the physician who conducts the autopsy. Although prenatal diagnostic testing and imaging are important and often highly informative, the neonatal autopsy plays a valuable role in evaluation of neonatal death. Neonatal autopsy can be very different from an adult autopsy for many reasons including the fact that diseases or conditions considered in adult death are often different from those in fetal death and the consideration that fetal health and development can be influenced by maternal health and the intrauterine environment (Désilets et al., 2011). An autopsy may be performed in two ways: full or limited. Autopsy involves removing organs from the body and the physical examination of the external body, internal organs, and placenta, as well as of representative tissue samples saved and tested. External evaluation may include photographs, X-ray, and MRI (Désilets et al., 2011). Tissue testing may include karyotype, viral studies, and microscopic staining. A full autopsy includes evaluation of the organs of the chest, abdomen, and brain. A limited autopsy is often dictated by the parents of the neonate and can place limitations on what can and cannot be evaluated and in what ways that evaluation can occur. For example, parents could state that they want evaluation of the "chest only" in a baby with a heart defect. Other parents may ask for only an examination of the external body of the baby.

Addressing the option of autopsy can be a difficult conversation. A provider must be sensitive while also providing all the necessary information for making the decision. There are many reasons a family might consider an autopsy, including determining the cause of death, identifying and characterizing congenital structural abnormalities, providing or refuting a diagnosis and possible recurrence risk, and management of future pregnancies, as well as potential opportunities for learning and research that may benefit other families (Désilets et al., 2011). It is important to note that if a family chooses to have an autopsy, this does not prevent them from spending time with the baby or having funeral or memorial services. Other families may choose not to complete an autopsy for other reasons: commonly, these include the feeling that the baby has suffered enough, assuming prenatal assessments were adequate, or cultural and religious beliefs (Désilets et al., 2011). For these families, sometimes a limited autopsy is a good option.

Palliative Care or Hospice

Palliative care refers to interventions used to relieve suffering and improve the quality of life for those with a disease using pain and symptom control as well as psychological, social, and spiritual support (Klick, Hauer, 2010). *Hospice* is the medical care and support received by those with terminal conditions nearing the end of life (Calhoun et al., 2006). Neonatal hospice and palliative care refer to these types of services when a fetus or newborn is diagnosed with a condition that will result in death. These two terms are often used synonymously. Neonatal services are often provided by a tertiary care center and are separate and unique from other forms of adult palliative care and hospice. These services can include counseling, birth planning, plans for the levels of care for the infant after birth, anticipatory grief preparation, funeral/service planning, and discussions regarding methods of bonding with the baby prior to birth and/or death (Calhoun et al., 2006). These services are usually offered at the time of diagnosis and can extend until a year after the death of the infant (Calhoun et al., 2006; Klick, Hauer, 2010).

Support Referrals and Bereavement

An important part of genetic counseling is helping patients understand that they are not alone. One of the ways in which genetic counselors are uniquely positioned to help with this process is to provide resources for support, information, and advocacy. Advocacy groups can provide specific information regarding the genetic condition or anomaly, as well as unique perspectives on things like living with the condition, decision-making, and the like. Many advocacy groups will give patients the opportunity to meet with or contact people who have previously gone through what the patient might be experiencing. These groups are also typically geared toward families instead of health care professionals, which can provide unique perspectives not found anywhere else. It is important to note that not all advocacy groups are for all types of people. Some groups may be better suited for a patient with a certain set of values, while another may be better suited for a different set of values. For example, an advocacy group made up of families who elected to continue a pregnancy and elect palliative care may not be appropriate for a woman considering termination for the same condition. A genetic counselor can be very helpful in sorting through these different groups and guiding the patient toward those that are most aligned with her values and decisions (Uhlmann, 2009).

Support is particularly important in the perinatal setting because patients and their families are "grieving the wanted child" (Kolker, Burke, 1993; Ramdaney et al., 2015). Perinatal grief can be different from other types of loss because there is often a lack of social support and validation as well as social minimization of the loss when compared to traditionally accepted forms of loss (Lang et al., 2011; Kersting, Wagner, 2012). Grief after perinatal loss is sometimes called *disenfranchised grief* or *complicated grief* for these very reasons (Lang et al., 2011; Kersting, Wagner, 2012). Those who experience perinatal loss may also experience posttraumatic stress, depression, anxiety, and sleep difficulties (Hutti, 2005; Kersting, Wagner, 2012; Lang et al., 2011). Grief in the perinatal setting does not necessarily have to follow death. When patients receive unexpected news about their unborn baby, they grieve the loss of their hopes and dreams for that child, whether the baby will live or not (Bourguignon et al., 1999).

Those who experience perinatal loss differ from traditional grief in many ways. These can include intense feelings of guilt and self-blame, women feeling as if their bodies have failed them, and feelings of child envy that can make it a struggle to have contact with friends and family who have children or are pregnant (Kersting, Wagner,

2012). Perinatal loss is often sudden and unanticipated (Kersting, Wagner, 2012; Ramdaney et al., 2015), particularly in a society where parents expect successful and uncomplicated pregnancies (Badenhorst, Hughes, 2006). Parents have little or no direct life experiences with the baby they lost as they would with the death of any other close member of the family (Kersting, Wagner, 2012). Often there is no funeral or traditional mourning ritual, which can lead to others not acknowledging the loss (Kersting, Wagner, 2012; Lang et al., 2011). Those who experience perinatal loss often report feeling as if their medical provider minimized their loss and was not adequately supportive (Lang et al., 2011). Poor levels of support have been associated with prolonged grief (Badenhorst, Hughes, 2006).

Women who elect a termination have similar responses to their perinatal loss despite the loss itself being planned. No reports of differences in the grief process have been reported when compared to an unexpected loss (Kersting, Wagner, 2012). Women who terminated their pregnancy due to a genetic condition or anomaly reported being unprepared for the psychological consequences after the procedure (LaFarge, 2014; Ramdaney et al., 2015). Many women who choose termination often have the additional complication of societal disapproval or stigma because of their decision, which can compound the grieving process (Kersting, Wagner, 2012; LaFarge, 2014; Maguire et al., 2015; Ramdaney et al., 2015).

Regardless of the type of perinatal loss, women and their families who experience loss reported the need for additional support and resources during this time (Hutti, 2005; LaFarge et al., 2013; LaFarge, 2014; Ramdaney et al., 2015).

Conclusion

As an integral part of the multidisciplinary care team for a patient with a high-risk pregnancy, a perinatal genetic counselor will need to be familiar with the roles of other team members and how everyone works together to provide the patient with the best possible care. The perinatal counselor also needs to understand his or her specific role within this team, whether it is discussing pregnancy options or providing referrals for bereavement. Given a genetic counselor's specialized training, this role often includes providing the patient with education and support specific to her situation while integrating the patient's personal values and beliefs.

References

Adzick NS, Thom EA, Spong CY, Brock JW 3rd, Burrows PK, Johnson MP, Howell LJ, Farrell JA, Dabrowiak ME, Sutton LN, Gupta N, Tulipan NB, D'Alton ME, Farmer DL; MOMS Investigators. A randomized trial of prenatal versus postnatal repair of myelomeningocele. *N Engl J Med*. 2011 Mar 17;364(11):993–1004.

American Academy of Pediatrics. What is a Pediatric Geneticist? https://www.healthychildren.org/English/family-life/health-management/pediatric-specialists/Pages/What-is-a-Pediatric-Geneticist.aspx. Updated 11/15/2015. Accessed June 22, 2017.

American College of Obstetricians and Gynecologists and Society for Maternal–Fetal Medicine; Menard MK, Kilpatrick S, Saade G, Hollier LM, Joseph GF Jr, Barfield W, Callaghan W, Jennings J, Conry J. Levels of maternal care. *Am J Obstet Gynecol*. 2015 Mar;212(3):259–271.

American College of Obstetricians and Gynecologists. Frequently asked questions: FAQ043 Special procedures induced abortion. May 2015. https://www.acog.org/-/media/For-Patients/faq043.pdf. Accessed April 27 2016.

American College of Obstetricians and Gynecologists. Frequently asked questions FAQ168 Pregnancy choices: raising the baby, adoption, and abortion. February 2013. https://www.acog.org/~/media/For%20Patients/faq168.pdf. Access April 27 2017.

American College of Obstetricians and Gynecologists. Practice bulletin no. 143: Medical management of first-trimester abortion. *Obstet Gynecol*. 2014 Mar;123(3):676–692.

American College of Obstetricians and Gynecologists (ACOG) Committee on Genetics. ACOG practice bulletin no. 135: Second-trimester abortion. *Obstet Gynecol*. 2013 Jun;121(6):1394–1406.

Atrash HK, Hogue CJ. The effect of pregnancy termination on future reproduction. *Baillieres Clin Obstet Gynaecol.* 1990 Jun;4(2):391–405.

Ayres A, Johnson TR. Management of multiple pregnancy: prenatal care--part II. *Obstet Gynecol Surv.* 2005 Aug;60(8):538–549.

Badenhorst W, Hughes P. Psychological aspects of perinatal loss. *Best Pract Res Clin Obstet Gynaecol.* 2007 Apr;21(2):249–259.

Benachi A, Sarnacki S. Prenatal counselling and the role of the paediatric surgeon. *Semin Pediatr Surg.* 2014 Oct;23(5):240–243.

Bourguignon A, Briscoe B, Nemzer L. Genetic abortion: considerations for patient care. *J Perinat Neonatal Nurs.* 1999 Sep;13(2):47–58.

Calhoun BC, Napolitano P, Terry M, Bussey C, Hoeldtke NJ. Perinatal hospice. Comprehensive care for the family of the fetus with a lethal condition. *J Reprod Med.* 2003 May;48(5):343–348.

Colombani PM. What's new in pediatric surgery. *J Am Coll Surg.* 2003 Aug;197(2):278–284.

Davis AS, Chock VY, Hintz SR. Fetal centers and the role of the neonatologist in complex fetal care. *Am J Perinatol.* 2014 Aug;31(7):549–556.

Désilets V, Oligny LL; Genetics Committee of the Society of Obstetricians and Gynaecology Canada; Family Physicians Advisory Committee; Medico–Legal Committee of the SOGC. Fetal and perinatal autopsy in prenatally diagnosed fetal abnormalities with normal karyotype. *J Obstet Gynaecol Can.* 2011 Oct;33(10):1047–1057. Review.

Dickinson JE, Prime DK, Charles AK. The role of autopsy following pregnancy termination for fetal abnormality. *Aust N Z J Obstet Gynaecol.* 2007 Dec;47(6):445–449.

Gagnon A, Wilson RD, Allen VM, Audibert F, Blight C, Brock JA, Désilets VA, Johnson JA, Langlois S, Murphy-Kaulbeck L, Wyatt P; Society of Obstetricians and Gynaecologists of Canada. Evaluation of prenatally diagnosed structural congenital anomalies. *J Obstet Gynaecol Can.* 2009 Sep;31(9):875–881, 882–889.

Glenn OA, Coakley FV. MRI of the fetal central nervous system and body. *Clin Perinatol.* 2009 Jun;36(2):273–300, viii.

Hern WM, Zen C, Ferguson KA, Hart V, Haseman MV. Outpatient abortion for fetal anomaly and fetal death from 15–34 menstrual weeks' gestation: techniques and clinical management. *Obstet Gynecol.* 1993 Feb;81(2):301–306.

Hutti MH. Social and professional support needs of families after perinatal loss. *J Obstet Gynecol Neonatal Nurs.* 2005 Sep–Oct;34(5):630–638.

Jacobs AR, Dean G, Wasenda EJ, Porsch LM, Moshier EL, Luthy DA, Paul ME. Late termination of pregnancy for lethal fetal anomalies: a national survey of maternal-fetal medicine specialists. *Contraception.* 2015 Jan;91(1):12–18.

Kersting A, Wagner B. Complicated grief after perinatal loss. *Dialogues Clin Neurosci.* 2012 Jun;14(2):187–194. Review.

Klick JC, Hauer J. Pediatric palliative care. *Curr Probl Pediatr Adolesc Health Care.* 2010 Jul;40(6):120–151.

Kolker A, Burke BM. Grieving the wanted child: ramifications of abortion after prenatal diagnosis of abnormality. *Health Care Women Int.* 1993 Nov–Dec;14(6):513–526.

Kruse B, Poppema S, Creinin MD, Paul M. Management of side effects and complications in medical abortion. *Am J Obstet Gynecol.* 2000 Aug;183(2 Suppl):S65–75.

Kulier R, Kapp N, Gülmezoglu AM, Hofmeyr GJ, Cheng L, Campana A. Medical methods for first trimester abortion. *Cochrane Database Syst Rev.* 2011 Nov 9;(11):CD002855.

Lafarge C, Mitchell K, Fox P. Termination of pregnancy for fetal abnormality: a meta-ethnography of women's experiences. *Reprod Health Matters.* 2014 Nov;22(44):191–201.

Lafarge C, Mitchell K, Fox P. Women's experiences of coping with pregnancy termination for fetal abnormality. *Qual Health Res.* 2013 Jul;23(7):924–936.

Lang A, Fleiszer AR, Duhamel F, Sword W, Gilbert KR, Corsini-Munt S. Perinatal loss and parental grief: the challenge of ambiguity and disenfranchised grief. *Omega (Westport).* 2011;63(2):183–196.

Legendre CM, Moutel G, Drouin R, Favre R, Bouffard C. Differences between selective termination of pregnancy and fetal reduction in multiple pregnancy: a narrative review. *Reprod Biomed Online.* 2013 Jun;26(6):542–554.

Lohr PA, Hayes JL, Gemzell-Danielsson K. Surgical versus medical methods for second trimester induced abortion. *Cochrane Database Syst Rev.* 2008 Jan 23;(1):CD006714.

Maguire M, Light A, Kuppermann M, Dalton VK, Steinauer JE, Kerns JL. Grief after second-trimester termination for fetal anomaly: a qualitative study. *Contraception.* 2015 Mar;91(3):234–239.

Miller ES, Minturn L, Linn R, Weese-Mayer DE, Ernst LM. Stillbirth evaluation: a stepwise assessment of placental pathology and autopsy. *Am J Obstet Gynecol.* 2016 Jan;214(1):115.e1–6.

Peranteau WH, Adzick NS. Prenatal surgery for myelomeningocele. *Curr Opin Obstet Gynecol.* 2016 Apr;28(2):111–118.

Ramdaney A, Hashmi SS, Monga M, Carter R, Czerwinski J. Support desired by women following termination of pregnancy for a fetal anomaly. *J Genet Couns.* 2015 Dec;24(6):952–960.

Rogers L, Li J, Liu L, Balluz R, Rychik J, Ge S. Advances in fetal echocardiography: early imaging, three/four dimensional imaging, and role of fetal echocardiography in guiding early postnatal management of congenital heart disease. *Echocardiography.* 2013 Apr;30(4):428–438.

Rychik J, Ayres N, Cuneo B, Gotteiner N, Hornberger L, Spevak PJ, Van Der Veld M. American Society of Echocardiography guidelines and standards for performance of the fetal echocardiogram. *J Am Soc Echocardiogr.* 2004 Jul;17(7):803–810.

Sanapo L, Moon-Grady AJ, Donofrio MT. Perinatal and delivery management of infants with congenital heart disease. *Clin Perinatol.* 2016 Mar;43(1):55–71.

Sepulveda W, Wong AE, Sepulveda F, Martinez-Ten P, Ximenes R. Fetal magnetic resonance imaging and three-dimensional ultrasound in clinical practice: general aspects. *Best Pract Res Clin Obstet Gynaecol.* 2012 Oct;26(5):575–591.

Society for Maternal–Fetal Medicine (SMFM), Sciscione A, Berghella V, Blackwell S, Boggess K, Helfgott A, Iriye B, Keller J, Menard MK, O'Keeffe D, Riley L, Stone J. Society for maternal-fetal medicine (SMFM) special report: the maternal-fetal medicine subspecialists' role within a health care system. *Am J Obstet Gynecol.* 2014 Dec;211(6):607–616.

Stewart KS, Johnson MP, Quintero RA, Evans MI. Congenital abnormalities in twins: selective termination. *Curr Opin Obstet Gynecol.* 1997 Apr;9(2):136–139.

Sudhakaran N, Sothinathan U, Patel S. Best practice guidelines: fetal surgery. *Early Hum Dev.* 2012 Jan;88(1):15–19.

Uhlmann W. Thinking it all through: case preparation and management. In: Uhlmann, W, Schuette, J, and Yshar, B, eds. *A guide to genetic counseling.* Hoboken, NJ: John Wiley; 2009:71–131.

Wenstrom KD, Carr SR. Fetal surgery: principles, indications, and evidence. *Obstet Gynecol.* 2014 Oct;124(4):817–835.

Wildschut H, Both MI, Medema S, Thomee E, Wildhagen MF, Kapp N. Medical methods for mid-trimester termination of pregnancy. *Cochrane Database Syst Rev.* 2011 Jan 19;(1):CD005216.

Wimalasundera RC. Selective reduction and termination of multiple pregnancies. *Semin Fetal Neonatal Med.* 2010 Dec;15(6):327–335.

Wright C, Sibley CP, Baker PN. The role of fetal magnetic resonance imaging. *Arch Dis Child Fetal Neonatal Ed.* 2010 Mar;95(2):F137–141.

Yaron Y, Johnson KD, Bryant-Greenwood PK, Kramer RL, Johnson MP, Evans MI. Selective termination and elective reduction in twin pregnancies: 10 years experience at a single centre. *Hum Reprod.* 1998 Aug;13(8):2301–2304.

Yonke N, Leeman LM. First-trimester surgical abortion technique. *Obstet Gynecol Clin North Am.* 2013 Dec;40(4):647–670.

8

Assisted Reproductive Technology and Reproductive Options for the At-Risk Couple

Many patients seen in the perinatal setting are pregnant due to assisted reproductive technologies (ART), have questions about ART, or are couples or individuals at risk of having a child with an inherited condition and who may be eligible for in vitro fertilization (IVF) with preimplantation genetic diagnosis (PGD). This chapter will describe the basics of ART and reproductive options.

Reproductive Options for At-Risk Couples

Those with an increased risk of having a child with a genetic condition have several types of reproductive options: (1) avoiding pregnancy altogether, (2) undergoing prenatal diagnosis in a current pregnancy, and (3) preventing transmission of the genetic changes responsible for the condition to a child (Jones, Fallon, 2002). Avoidance of pregnancy can be achieved by a couple choosing to remain childless or adopting a nonbiological child. Prenatal diagnosis (as discussed in Chapter 4) allows the couple to achieve pregnancy through their preferred method and complete testing on that pregnancy, and make decisions based on test results. The last method, preventing the transmission of the genetic condition to a child, may be accomplished in two ways. The first is to use a gamete (egg or sperm) donor or embryo donor to achieve pregnancy. *Donor gametes* allow for one parent to be genetically related to the child while both still experience the pregnancy and birth process. *Donor embryos* allow for the pregnancy and birth experience while allowing both parents to choose not to contribute their genetic material to the child. The second is to complete IVF with preimplantation genetic testing of the embryo prior to implantation (see the section "Preimplantation Genetic Testing"). Each of these options will be perceived differently by different types of patients and families (Jones, Fallon, 2002). It is important to note that, aside from a couple choosing to remain childless, none of these options will guarantee the birth of a healthy child. All options should be presented to an at-risk couple, and the decision should be guided by their personal values and beliefs.

Assisted Reproductive Techniques

Various types of techniques are available to assist with reproduction. Most of these techniques are not used for the at-risk genetic patient but may be encountered in the perinatal clinic.

In *ovarian stimulation*, the ovaries are medically stimulated to produce multiple follicles that lead to the availability of multiple oocytes for fertilization (ESHRE Capri Workshop Group, 2009). This is often used in women who do not ovulate on their own or in conjunction with other techniques. Ovarian stimulation increases the likelihood for multiple gestations.

Intrauterine insemination (IUI) is a method used in couples who are considered subfertile or in those who choose to use a sperm donor because they are at increased risk or are of the same sex as their partner. This technique involves collection of sperm, processing of sperm to remove plasma, resuspension into culture media, and deposition of the suspension directly into the uterus, peritoneum, or fallopian tube (ESHRE Capri Workshop Group, 2009). IUI can be done in conjunction with or without ovarian stimulation (ESHRE Capri Workshop Group, 2009).

IVF is a method of assisted reproduction in which sperm and egg are combined outside of the body in a laboratory, and one or more embryos are transferred into the uterus for implantation. IVF involves ovarian stimulation, egg retrieval, fertilization, embryo culture, and embryo transfer. The process of ovarian stimulation is the same as described earlier, but the goal is usually many more mature follicles. This is because some of the eggs retrieved will not fertilize or produce a viable embryo. Egg retrieval is the process by which the mature oocytes are surgically removed. This is done with a transvaginal ultrasound-guided needle inserted into the follicles; the needle is connected to a suction device. After egg retrieval, the eggs are examined microscopically for quality and maturity. Mature oocytes are placed in culture, and prepared sperm is either placed directly in the culture with the egg for typical fertilization or is introduced by intracyotplasmic sperm injection (ICSI). ICSI is a process by which a single sperm is injected directly into the mature oocyte. The fertilized oocyte is then cultured for 5–6 days until it becomes a multicelled embryo, called a *blastocyst*. Embryo(s) can be transferred into the uterus between 1 and 6 days after egg retrieval. Unused embryos at this stage may be frozen for future use (cryopreservation) (Society for Assisted Reproductive Technology, 2017). IVF is necessary to complete preimplantation genetic testing as well as for those choosing to use donor eggs to achieve pregnancy.

Preimplantation Genetic Testing

Preimplantation genetic testing refers to the ability to analyze the genetic composition of an embryo produced by IVF prior to implanting that embryo into the uterus (Practice Committee of the ASRM, 2007). There are two methods of testing available: *preimplantation genetic screening (PGS)* and *preimplantation genetic diagnosis (PGD)*. These testing options allow for an increased probability that a subsequent child will be free of the particular genetic condition screened for (Audibert et al., 2009;Dahdouh, 2015).

Preimplantation Genetic Screening

PGS is the type of test used when both parents are presumed to have typical chromosomes and their embryos are screened for aneuploidy (ASRM, 2007). PGS is typically accomplished by allowing the fertilized embryo to grow into a blastocyst, by day 5 or 6, and subsequently removing 5–10 cells from the trophectoderm (the outermost layer of cells). Other stages of embryo development may be used for biopsy, such as the cleavage stage (3-day embryo), or a biopsy of the oocyte polar body. These techniques are not the typical method of choice in the United States, given that an oocyte polar body provides only information about maternally inherited chromosomal conditions, and cleavage-stage biopsy has been shown to have detrimental effects on the development of the embryo (Dahdouh et al., 2015; Lu et al., 2016). The biopsied cells are then screened for aneuploidy (see Figure 8.1).

The embryo is typically frozen while genetic testing is completed. The most common genetic screening method is a microarray analysis, using either single nucleotide polymorphism (SNP)-based or comparative technologies (ASRM, 2007; Dahdouh et al., 2015). Microarray analysis performed on embryo samples will not have the same depth of coverage as a microarray performed on fetal or blood samples. Microarray analysis allows for analysis of the entire chromosome complement as well as lower levels of copy number changes. The limitations of microarray analysis may include the inability of the testing platform to find balanced translocations and mosaicism, as well as amplification bias of the normal chromosome complement (Dahdouh et al., 2015). Other methods exist for analyzing the trophectoderm cells including quantitative polymerase chain reaction (qPCR) and fluorescence in situ hybridization (FISH). FISH will only be able to provide information about a small number of chromosomes given that probes are not available for all 24 chromosomes, but it can be useful in identifying unbalanced translocations (ASRM, 2007; Audibert et al., 2009; Dahdouh et al., 2015). qPCR can typically be performed rapidly, within 4 hours, which allows for the use of a fresh embryo in the uterine

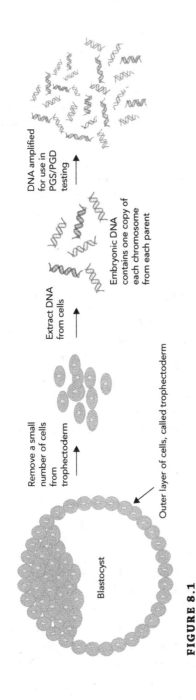

FIGURE 8.1

Trophectoderm biopsy and preimplantation genetic screening.

transfer. This technology amplifies two sequences on each arm of each chromosome; these are then quantified to allow comparison across the genome. This technique uses a direct sample, which may limit the amplification bias seen in microarray analysis. This technology is limited by the number of embryos that can be analyzed at once and the failure rate of results from direct sample (Dahdouh et al., 2015). It is important to note that PGS is a screening test and cannot guarantee that the embryo is free of chromosome anomalies. PGS may be useful in women older than 35, in those with multiple pregnancy losses with normal parental karyotype, or in those with previous unsuccessful embryo transfers (ASRM, 2007; Audibert et al., 2009). However, PGS has not been shown to improve live birth rates (ASRM, 2007).

Preimplantation Genetic Diagnosis

PGD is the term used when testing an embryo for a single-gene disorder or chromosome rearrangement that one or both parents carry to prevent that specific mutation(s) from being transmitted to a future child (ASRM, 2007). These disorders can be autosomal recessive, autosomal dominant, or X-linked (ASRM, 2007; Audibert et al., 2009). PGD is similar to PGS in that it requires a biopsy of cells from the developing embryo, which most often occurs at the blastocyst stage of development. These cells will then be used for genetic testing while the embryo is frozen to arrest development. Oocyte polar body biopsy may be used when the gene of interest is X-linked (ASRM, 2007; Basille et al., 2009). Once an embryo is identified as being free from the mutation(s) of interest, they can be selected for implantation while those that are found to carry the mutation(s) of interest will not be used.

The testing approach for PGD is more complicated than for PGS. In order for a couple to be eligible for PGD, a condition-causing mutation(s) must be identified in the parents within the gene of interest, called a *familial mutation*. Therefore, parents must complete genetic testing themselves prior to pursuing PGD (ASRM, 2007). If a mutation cannot be identified in a parent, PGD may not be able to be performed.

Although in post-natal testing, direct mutation analysis is adequate, in PGD an additional method is necessary to ensure the most accurate diagnosis. Once the mutations in the parents are known, a process called *linkage-analysis* is typically completed (Reproductive Genetics Institute [RGI], 2012). Linkage analysis is used to determine the likelihood that two or more genetic sequences will be passed on together. Two genetic sequences that are closer to each other on the same chromosome are more likely to be inherited together than two sequences that are further apart, due to naturally occurring recombination events. The genetic sequences surrounding the mutation of interest are evaluated to determine if any of them are close enough to be inherited together or as a "linked" unit. The surrounding genetic sequences in this situation are called the *linked markers*. Linked markers are specific to each genetic condition, as well as to the individuals in the family. Each family will have a unique number and location of linked markers (Jorde et al., 2010; Nussbaum et al., 2007; RGI, 2012). Linked markers must be located prior to PGD testing of the embryo. Locating linked markers requires blood samples both from healthy individuals in the family as well as from those who are either affected or are known carriers of the familial mutation in the gene of interest. The markers located closest to the mutation of interest are compared between the healthy individuals and the carriers/affected individuals throughout the generations. By determining which markers are always inherited with the copy of the mutation of interest and which are always associated with the unaffected copy of the gene, the laboratory can determine if the gene mutation of interest is present in the embryo even if *allele dropout* (ADO) occurs (explained next) (Collins, 2013; RGI, 2012). Linkage analysis allows the laboratory to use more than just the single mutation of interest to determine if the embryo is carrying the familial mutation (ASRM, 2007; Collins, 2013; RGI, 2012). See Figure 8.2 for a diagram of the linkage analysis process.

ADO is a phenomenon that can occur when the amount of a DNA sample needs to be increased (amplified). There are only very small amounts of DNA available from the few cells collected during

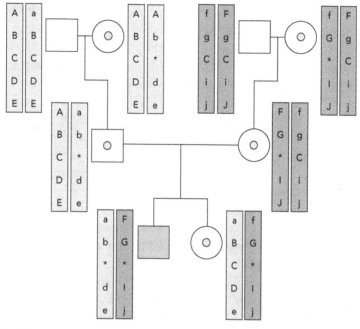

FIGURE 8.2

Linkage analysis for preimplantation genetic diagnosis.

the embryo biopsy, and this amount would not be enough to be usable for testing (ASRM, 2007; Audibert et al., 2009). DNA amplification by PCR requires the separation into single strands of the two helical strands of DNA that contain the gene of interest from each chromosome (maternal and paternal copies in the embryo). Separation is followed by the use of a highly specific strand of manufactured DNA, called a *primer*, that attaches itself to the single-stranded DNA near the gene of interest. The primer acts as a starting point to make a copy of the DNA it has attached to (Blais et al., 2015). The result is now doubled, or four, strands of DNA that contain the gene of interest. This process is repeated 30–40 times, which results in billions of copies of the DNA that contains the gene of interest. See Figure 8.3 for a diagram of PCR.

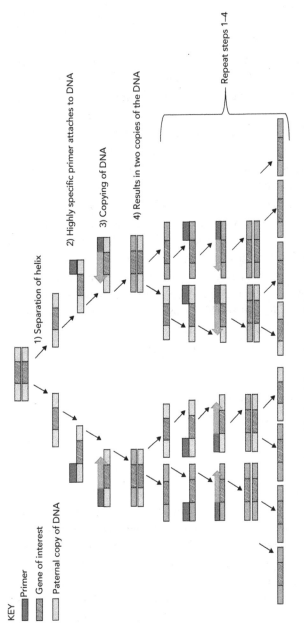

KEY

■ Primer
■ Gene of interest
▨ Paternal copy of DNA

1) Separation of helix

2) Highly specific primer attaches to DNA

3) Copying of DNA

4) Results in two copies of the DNA

Repeat steps 1–4

Repeat 30–40x = billions of copies of the gene of interest

*Of note, this diagram is only showing the paternal copy of the gene of interest being copied. This is also occurring with the maternal copy of the gene of interest simultaneously.

FIGURE 8.3

Polymerase chain reaction (PCR) diagram.

ADO occurs when only one copy of the gene of interest amplifies (from only one chromosome) instead of both copies (one from each chromosome) (ASRM, 2007; Blais et al., 2015; Collins, 2013; RGI, 2012). Because amplification uses a highly specific primer to start the process of copying the DNA, if that primer does not attach itself to the DNA in the first place (due to random genetic changes in the DNA), then that particular copy of the gene of interest will not amplify while the copy on the other chromosome will. This will result in the misrepresentation of the presence or absence of a specific mutation in the gene of interest (Blais et al., 2015). See Figure 8.4. For example, if the gene of interest is *CFTR* for cystic fibrosis and the father has a random DNA change at the site where the primer would normally attach, then the paternal copy of the *CFTR* gene would not be amplified, and only the maternal copy would. Thus, when the mutations in *CFTR* were screened, the embryo could appear as a carrier for cystic fibrosis instead of being affected. If linkage is completed, then the laboratory can look at the marker that is linked to the paternal copy of the *CFTR* gene to determine if the embryo inherited the mutation of interest or not, even when ADO has occurred. This can reduce the likelihood of a misdiagnosis or inconclusive results due to ADO (ASRM, 2007; Collins, 2013; RGI, 2012).

It is important to note the limitations of PGD. Not all familial mutations will have adequate linked markers available for analysis, and recombination can never be completely ruled out (RGI, 2012). There are occasions where there are not enough family members available to set linkage (Collins, 2013), and setting linkage can be difficult when the parent has a *de novo* mutation. Not all embryos will have a conclusive diagnosis after analysis. There is no guarantee that there will be a healthy embryo available for transfer, meaning that all the embryos tested might be affected. PGD cannot rule out other types of genetic conditions or birth defects not related to the condition being tested (RGI, 2012). As such, once a pregnancy is achieved, prenatal diagnosis should still be offered to confirm the PGD results (ASRM, 2007; Basille et al., 2009).

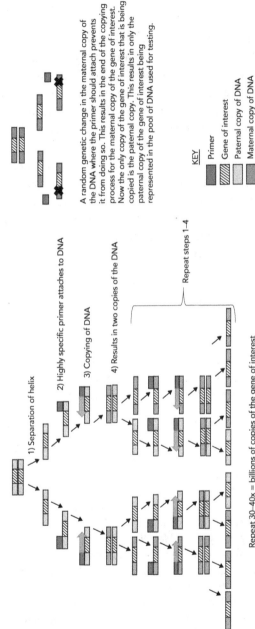

1) Separation of helix

2) Highly specific primer attaches to DNA

3) Copying of DNA

4) Results in two copies of the DNA

Repeat steps 1–4

A random genetic change in the maternal copy of the DNA where the primer should attach prevents it from doing so. This results in the end of the copying process for the maternal copy of the gene of interest. Now the only copy of the gene of interest that is being copied is the paternal copy. This results in only the paternal copy of the gene of interest being represented in the pool of DNA used for testing.

KEY

Primer
Gene of interest
Paternal copy of DNA
Maternal copy of DNA

Repeat 30–40x = billions of copies of the gene of interest

FIGURE 8.4

Allele drop-out.

Conclusion

ART will not be a part of every perinatal genetic counseling session. However, its use is increasing, and many of the patients seen in a perinatal clinic will have used these techniques. This overview provides the perinatal genetic counselor with general knowledge about ART technologies used by those of their patients being seen for discussion of screening and diagnostic options. It also discusses the use of preimplantation testing and acknowledges its complexity. Sometimes the perinatal genetic counselor is the first person to discuss the existence of these options for an at-risk couple to increase their chance for a healthy child. Many reproductive clinics have genetic counselors on staff who specialize in ART techniques. However, many other reproductive clinics do not employ genetic counselors, and patients will be seen by a perinatal counselor once a pregnancy is achieved.

References

Audibert F, Wilson RD, Allen V, Blight C, Brock JA, Désilets VA, Gagnon A, Johnson JA, Langlois S, Wyatt P; Genetics Committee. Preimplantation genetic testing. *J Obstet Gynaecol Can.* 2009 Aug;31(8):761–775.

Basille C, Frydman R, El Aly A, Hesters L, Fanchin R, Tachdjian G, Steffann J, LeLorc'h M, Achour-Frydman N. Preimplantation genetic diagnosis: state of the art. *Eur J Obstet Gynecol Reprod Biol.* 2009 Jul;145(1):9–13.

Blais J, Lavoie SB, Giroux S, Bussières J, Lindsay C, Dionne J, Laroche M, Giguère Y, Rousseau F. Risk of misdiagnosis due to allele dropout and false-positive PCR artifacts in molecular diagnostics: analysis of 30,769 genotypes. *J Mol Diagn.* 2015 Sep;17(5):505–514.

Collins SC. Preimplantation genetic diagnosis: technical advances and expanding applications. *Curr Opin Obstet Gynecol.* 2013 Jun;25(3):201–206.

Dahdouh EM, Balayla J, Audibert F; Genetics Committee; Wilson RD, Audibert F, Brock JA, Campagnolo C, Carroll J, Chong K, Gagnon

A, Johnson JA, MacDonald W, Okun N, Pastuck M, Vallée-Pouliot K. Technical update: preimplantation genetic diagnosis and screening. *J Obstet Gynaecol Can.* 2015 May;37(5):451–463.

ESHRE Capri Workshop Group. Intrauterine insemination. *Hum Reprod Update.* 2009 May–Jun;15(3):265–277.

Jones SL, Fallon LA. Reproductive options for individuals at risk for transmission of a genetic disorder. *J Obstet Gynecol Neonatal Nurs.* 2002 Mar-Apr;31(2):193–199.

Jorde L, Carey J, Bamshad M. (2010). *Medical genetics.* 4th ed. Philadelphia: Mosby Elsevier.

Lu L, Lv B, Huang K, Xue Z, Zhu X, Fan G. Recent advances in preimplantation genetic diagnosis and screening. *J Assist Reprod Genet.* 2016 Sep;33(9):1129–1134.

Nussbaum R, McInnes R, Willard H. (2007). *Thompson & Thompson genetics in medicine.* 7th ed. Philadelphia: Saunders Elsevier.

Practice Committee of the Society for Assisted Reproductive Technology; Practice Committee of the American Society for Reproductive Medicine. Preimplantation genetic testing: a Practice Committee opinion. *Fertil Steril.* 2007 Dec;88(6): 1497–1504.

Reproductive Genetics Institute (RGI). Preimplantation Genetic Diagnosis (PGD): single gene disorders. *A Patient Guide.* December 2012:463–471.

Society for Assisted Reproductive Technology. A patient's guide to assisted reproductive technology. 1996–2017. http://www.sart.org/patients/a-patients-guide-to-assisted-reproductive-technology/general-information/. Accessed March 2017.

9

Common Perinatal Genetic Counseling Situations

Prenatal counselors are often faced with challenging circumstances, complex counseling situations, and ethical dilemmas. Some of these situations are unique to the perinatal setting while others are more generalizable to all areas of genetic counseling and testing. Counselors are uniquely qualified to respond to these situations given their skills in giving difficult news, facilitating the decision-making process, and working with patients and their families, as well as being aware of and helping patients to incorporate religious and cultural perspectives. Numerous published materials are available to assist in the development of these genetic counseling skills, and the National Society of Genetic Counselors (NSGC) code of ethics is available to guide counselors when faced with ethical dilemmas. Additionally, genetic counselors will need to follow the specific regulations and rules dictated by the institutions at which they are employed. Rather than reiterate those concepts here, this chapter will highlight common situations that a perinatal counselor may experience and should be aware of.

Pregnancy Termination

Needless to say, the option and the act of pregnancy termination are controversial: some people are always against it, others are pro-choice and may elect this for themselves, and others only accept this as an option in specific situations such as rape, when there is a grave fetal defect, in cases of incest, or when the life of the mother is at risk. It has long been stressed in the practice of genetic counseling that the counselor should take a nondirective approach to this issue, with an emphasis placed on patient autonomy. Therefore, regarding pregnancy termination, we recommend supporting a patient in the choice she decides to make. However, this may not always be simple, and, in the process of working with patients, specific situations may arise that complicate matters.

Misinterpreted Intent

A health care provider who presents the choice of a pregnancy termination should choose his words carefully. Although it is likely that the provider has the intent to provide complete information of all reproductive options, some patients may perceive that this option is being specifically recommended just simply by raising it as an option. If the patient is against this option, it can cause stress in the patient–provider relationship. We recommend beginning a discussion on termination with a statement that introduces intent so that patients are aware that you are not recommending termination; rather, you are simply introducing all options, and you will support them in their decisions, whatever those may be.

Patient–Provider Conflict

A health care provider comes with his or her own values, biases, and cultural and religious beliefs. Therefore, the provider may not agree with pregnancy termination in general or for the specific reason that a patient is electing to complete a pregnancy termination. For example, a provider might have a conflict with a patient electing a pregnancy termination after identification of a mild or adult-onset condition, a patient pursuing a late-term abortion (>24 weeks gestation), or a couple electing a termination for a pregnancy identified to not be affected with a condition such as hearing loss or achondroplasia. Although a health care provider has the right to object to authorize or perform certain lawful medical services, it is argued that it is still essential to provide patients with all their options, be respectful of patients' choices, and assist them in making a referral to another health care provider if necessary (Cowley, 2017).

Incidental Findings

An *incidental finding* is an observation or result of potential clinical significance identified about a patient, couple, or their fetus that is unrelated to the indication for testing, was not intended to be discovered by a particular genetic test, or is discovered in a healthy subject (Westerfield et al., 2014). Incidental findings that are commonly discussed in prenatal genetic counseling include misattributed paternity, discovery of consanguinity, and identifying a patient or fetus with an unexpected condition or health risk. If the testing being pursued has the potential for identifying incidental findings, the patient should be warned of this possibility as part of the pretest informed consent process.

Misattributed Paternity

Misattributed paternity, also known as *mistaken paternity* or *nonpaternity*, is a situation in which the presumed father of a fetus or child is found not to be the biological father. Studies estimate that the rate of misattributed paternity ranges from 2% to 3% (Voracek et al., 2008). In some cases, this may be known before genetic testing takes place, and, in these situations, patients may even request prenatal paternity testing. Various companies offer prenatal paternity testing either by cell-free DNA (cfDNA) testing or by testing amniotic fluid or chorionic villi. Alternatively, testing can be pursued after birth. However, if this information is not known and is found incidentally after completing genetic testing, it can create a complicated situation for the counselor regarding how to disclose the information, and may subsequently result in a significant negative impact on the family. Different approaches have been argued regarding how the health care provider should approach this situation. Perhaps there is no "correct way," but options include disclosing only relevant genetic information while withholding misattributed paternity when possible or, if not possible, warning the mother first prior to disclosing the information (Tozzo et al., 2014).

Discovery of Consanguinity

Approximately 10% of couples are estimated to be related as second cousins or closer for the global population; this occurs most commonly in sub-Saharan Africa; the Middle East; and west, central, and south Asia; and less commonly in the United States (Bittles, Black, 2010). Although there are many people who knowingly and willingly enter these relationships given cultural, economic, and religious reasons, some have been forced into the relationship (e.g., mother is a minor or intellectually disabled) or a couple may be completely unaware of their biological relationship. The identification of consanguinity can be difficult to discuss with families when discovered incidentally. This is in part due to the potential adverse health outcomes for the child, legal implications for the parent(s), and social stigma perceived by the family. Guidelines exist about how laboratories should report this incidental finding to the clinician (Rehder et al., 2013) but little is published to guide clinicians in the disclosure of this information to patients. If there is suspected or confirmed abuse, clinicians have a duty to report cases and should follow protocols and laws regulated by their institution and state.

Identification of an Incidental Condition

Testing a fetus has the potential to identify an incidental condition such as an adult-onset disease that will not affect the child in the newborn period or childhood, will not alter pregnancy management, and may have unknown severity for later life. If such an adult-onset condition is identified in a fetus, it may indicate that one of the parents has the same condition and perhaps has not yet developed symptoms (ACOG no. 581). Although some patients will want to test a fetus specifically for known adult-onset condition in the family, when found incidentally, this can be a surprise for the couple, leaving them with worry for their own and their child's future health. Another potential situation occurs when an incidental condition is discovered by carrier testing. Instead of identifying carrier status, a patient may learn that he or she is actually affected with the condition. The counselor must be aware of the possibility of identification of incidental conditions, include this possibility during pretest counseling, and make appropriate referrals when necessary.

Privacy and Confidentiality

Privacy is a person's control over the circumstances, timing, and extent to which they share of themselves, and it refers to their right to limit access to their personal self (i.e., identifying information, personal thoughts, and lab results) by others. *Confidentiality* is the process of protecting and maintaining another individual's privacy. Laws require health care providers to maintain the confidentiality of a patient's health information. Although seemingly a simple concept, there are times when this may be difficult.

Genetics Is a Family Affair

Most medical information pertains primarily to an individual, but genetics has both individual and familial implications and thus genetic testing might indicate that the patient's family members are also at risk. Therefore, counselors may find themselves working with multiple people in the same family. In general, a medical release form is needed for a health care provider to access and utilize information from other family members. Additionally, a health care provider cannot notify other family members of their risk. Instead, we can educate our patients to speak to their family members about risks and encourage them to share genetic testing results. This is not always simple. Families have many different dynamics, including being secretive with their health history or estrangement or tense relationships. In addition, a patient may not understand the implications of genetic findings for other family members and may not perceive a need to disclose this information to others (Wiseman et al., 2010). Specifically sharing with the patient how results could impact other family members, suggesting they share their test results, and discussing options to inform family members, may empower the patient to provide this information to his or her family.

Secret Information

People don't always share all of their health history or reproductive history with everyone, including their current partners or other family members. This information may, however, be documented in their records. Ultimately, health care providers have the responsibility to protect their patients' information. Because patients often come to genetic counseling with others, there is the potential to accidentally disclose this information without the patient wanting it to be shared. For example, a common situation encountered in the perinatal field is a secret pregnancy termination or miscarriage. To avoid accidentally disclosing this information, a health care provider should ask if it is permissible to discuss pregnancy and medical histories in front of others. Careful phrasing of questions can allow the patient to provide desired information. For example, rather than asking about a pregnancy termination or miscarriage, a provider might ask, "How many pregnancies have you had, regardless of the outcome?" and "Were these full term, preterm, miscarriages, pregnancy terminations, or ectopic pregnancies?" This allows the patient to provide the information without the provider sharing confidential information.

Working with Couples

Many patients seen in the perinatal setting present as a couple unit. Each individual in a relationship has the potential to bring different values, beliefs, and preferences to the counseling session, and each couple will be unique in how they work through conflict and make joint decisions. As a counselor working with couples, it is important to consider both individuals and how the couple prefers to make decisions.

Couples in Conflict

When making decisions about a pregnancy, many expectant parents turn to each other for emotional support, deliberate the implications, and reach an agreement for a decision or action to be pursued. However, it is not uncommon for couples to differ in their opinions about what testing options to pursue or how to manage a pregnancy. If there is a perceived or actual disagreement, this creates a significant amount of decisional conflict for patients (Muller, Cameron, 2016). Most of the time when conflict exists a resolution can be reached, either by a compromise or for one to concede to the other's preferred choice. Possible ideas to facilitate this process are to have the couple consider each other's viewpoint; discuss worst-case and best-case scenarios with either choice; encourage seeking help and advice from others, including family, counselors, or religious leaders; and to consider taking more time to discuss the options prior to making a decision. As health care providers, we can assist couples in these conflicts, but ultimately the person seeking testing is the patient and the one you have an obligation to.

"It's Not My Body"

Occasionally, a patient will request her or his partner's opinion about whatever option is being presented. For example, perhaps a patient is deciding whether to pursue screening or diagnostic testing for a chromosome abnormality and asks his or her partner for their opinion. Many times, the reply is "it's not my body" or "it's your body," which implies that the patient and not the partner is responsible for the decision. This is often stated with the intent to be supportive and is not usually intentionally dismissive—but it may perceived in that way. Although this may work for some couples and be preferred in some situations, other patients are struggling to make decisions, want a shared responsibility for the decision, or value the other person's opinion and want to weigh it into their decision. Assessing the patient's reaction and exploring his or her desire for an opinion while at the same time identifying the underlying reason for the statement from the partner may be appropriate.

Dealing with Uncertainty

Prenatal counselors are often faced with couples experiencing situations of uncertainty. When there are high levels of uncertainty, genetic counselors should address the lack of available information, provide information that is available in a balanced manner, and then help the patient identify effective coping strategies to manage that uncertainty.

Fetal Diagnosis and Prognosis

Perhaps the most common situation of uncertainty is when a fetus has been identified with an ultrasound finding(s), but no diagnosis is identified after testing. Needless to say prenatal genetic testing has limitations and further testing after birth may be necessary before a diagnosis is determined. Even after birth, a diagnosis may not be established. Without a diagnosis, counseling on prognosis and recurrence risk becomes difficult and may not be possible. Even in the presence of a known diagnosis, the prognosis of a fetus may also be uncertain. Some conditions are rare, with limited to no information available to use for reference. Prognosis may even be difficult to determine with certainty in commonly understood conditions such as Down syndrome, given the significant degree of variability in each individual. Although the literature can be reviewed to obtain natural history information as well as taking the patient's unique clinical situation into account, determining the prognosis is not always possible.

Family History

A family history reflects the combined influences of shared genetic, behavioral, and environmental factors in families. Although, in 2004, the US Surgeon General launched the Family History Public Health Initiative (US Department of Health and Human Services, 2004) to increase discussions and awareness of the importance of family health history, it is not uncommon for a patient to present with limited or no information. For example, a patient who was adopted into a family may lack relevant history or, in some situations, have no records at all regarding his or her biological family. Alternatively, a patient may know a family member has "a condition" but may lack information on the specific diagnosis or if testing had been completed. Another common scenario is a patient who is fully informed on the history of a family member, and, despite all testing and evaluations, the affected family member lacks a clear diagnosis. Without more information, recurrence risks and implications to the patient's pregnancy may be uncertain and testing options limited. We recommend, when possible, encouraging patients to collect more information, making yourself available when more is known, and following the testing guidelines available.

Complex Conditions

Many prospective parents' concerns and questions are in regards to conditions that may have a familial predisposition but for which there are no defined inheritance patterns. Conditions that may fall into this category include bipolar disorder, schizophrenia, multiple sclerosis, asthma, diabetes, epilepsy, and heart disease. Although some common conditions may be monogenic, the vast majority will be multifactorial. Given this, a person with a family history has an increased risk of being affected or of having children affected, but that risk has to be estimated using the empirical data available. Given that empirical data may be limited and testing is not readily available to determine who will be affected or not, this can leave parents feeling a significant degree of uncertainty.

Variants of Uncertain Significance

A variant of uncertain significance (VUS) is a finding that cannot be unequivocally classified as benign or clinically significant (Kearney et al., 2011). This sort of finding in a fetus leads to a complex situation for the health care provider who must interpret and counsel about the potential clinical consequences of the variant. A clinical example to illustrate this point is a fetus identified with a VUS after completing a microarray on an amniocentesis sample. In this example, if the significance is unknown, further testing of parents may be considered. Testing may reveal the finding to be inherited from one parent or be *de novo* in the fetus. If inherited and the parent is phenotypically normal, this may mean that the variant is benign or because it has reduced penetrance. For example, a deletion with variable penetrance and associated with an increased risk of autism that is inherited from an apparently healthy mother leads to uncertainty about how the child will actually present. Will the child develop autism or have a presentation similar to its mother?

Fetal Sex Disclosure

Historically, patients learn the sex of their developing baby at the 20-week anatomy scan. Now, with the option of cfDNA screening, diagnostic testing methods, and preimplantation genetic screening (PGS) of embryos, patients have the opportunity to discover this information earlier in pregnancy or even choose the sex of their baby, in the case of PGS. Although seemingly simple, this introduces unique situations for the perinatal counselor to consider.

Patient's Desire to Know or Not

Although studies and experience suggest that most patients and their families want to know the sex of their baby (Maaji et al., 2010; Shukar-Ud-Din et al., 2013), it is becoming an increasingly popular option to wait until the baby is born or to receive this information secretly so a gender reveal party can be organized by a friend or family member. Given this, we recommend asking if this information is desired and how the patient wants to receive it. Clearly documenting the patient's desire and following the patient's request is very important because you don't want to be the person who tells them the sex if they had hoped for a surprise.

Testing May Reveal Sex Chromosome Abnormalities

Some patients will not want to know the fetal sex but, at the same time, will pursue testing that may identify sex chromosome abnormalities (SCAs). SCAs are among the most frequently occurring chromosome abnormalities, seen in about 25% of all chromosomal abnormalities detected by amniocentesis with an overall incidence of approximately 1 in 400 (Crandall et al., 1980; Nielsen, Wohlert, 1991). These conditions are complex to counsel on given that they typically have a milder presentation with few serious implications but may have the potential to be clinically significant. If a patient has requested not to know the fetal sex, she should be warned that should an SCA be identified, then the sex of the baby would be disclosed by sharing the condition identified. The patient should also be warned that the implications of a SCA may be mild and that this information may therefore be shared without a need for immediate medical management alterations.

Disorders Affecting a Specific Sex

If a patient is a carrier of an X-linked disorder (e.g., male at risk for X-linked hydrocephalus) or the baby is at-risk for a condition that can affect a particular sex differently (e.g., congenital adrenal hyperplasia may result in virilization of affected females), then discovering the fetal sex is often not only wanted, but also may change the management of the pregnancy. Patient's known to be at-risk for these conditions may pursue testing to determine the fetal sex (e.g., through cfDNA, fluorescence in situ hybridization [FISH], or chromosomes from chorionic villus sampling [CVS] or amniocentesis) prior to deciding if further testing for the condition of interest will be completed.

Testing Only for Sex

It is not uncommon to have a patient who is primarily interested in the fetal sex and may be pursuing testing solely for this reason. Testing options available clinically do not include a "sex only" option. A patient choosing to pursue testing for sex information should be informed that testing has the potential to identify risks or diagnose a pregnancy with a chromosome abnormality and is not designed for sex determination alone.

Fetal Sex May Be "Difficult News"

Although most patients will tell you they just want a healthy child, some are also hoping either secretly or overtly for a child of a particular sex. Perhaps they have a preference given cultural, economic, social, or genetic risk reasons. Regardless of what is motivating their desire, the fetal sex results may be perceived as "difficult news" and be received with feelings of grief and sadness. It is important to be aware of this possibility.

Patient Questions

Genetic counselors are taught to begin a session by *contracting*. This is the process of creating a mutual agenda for the session and includes both explaining what the provider plans to discuss and eliciting the patient's expectations of the session as well as her questions or concerns. Patients often come with specific questions, and, although most are straightforward and can be answered easily, there will be times where they are more complicated to answer.

"What Would You Do?"

Ideas and perceptions about risks, benefits, worst-case scenarios, and all other implications of a choice will vary from person to person. For example, a patient with a high risk of a chromosome abnormality on cfDNA screening who is deciding to do an amniocentesis to confirm results may have very different reactions to this option compared to another patient. Perhaps she would elect to terminate a pregnancy that is affected. Perhaps she is most worried about losing a pregnancy, regardless of whether the fetus has a chromosome abnormality or not. Although many patients know what the best option is for them, when faced with a decision that is particularly difficult the patient may want to know what you, the provider, would do in the same situation. Perhaps they feel that you, as an educated provider, would make a better decision or they want validation for the choice they feel is correct. Perhaps they want to be directed and do not want to take responsibility for the choice. Regardless of the motivation behind this question, there is no "correct choice" that will fit every individual.

When asked this question, it may be important to assess the intent behind the question so that this can be addressed. For example, if the patient actually wants validation for what she is choosing, this can be handled by acknowledging her choice and its appropriateness for her. Alternatively, a counselor may want to make a general statement about the variability in decisions that can be made and how any single decision will not fit everyone. Another option is to acknowledge the difficult decision and to suggest that you, as a provider, would do what the patient is doing. That is, you would collect all the necessary information; discuss the options with other individuals, such as a spouse or partner; and then make the best decision based on your own values, preferences, and perceptions of the situation.

When You Don't Know the Answer

Although it is imperative to be prepared in genetic counseling sessions and to anticipate possible questions that will arise, it is impossible to know the answer to everything. Occasionally, patients will ask about a condition that you have never heard of or ask a question that would be better answered by a different provider (e.g., OB provider). In these cases, if it is information about a condition or test that is unknown to you, be honest and offer to research this information for the patient. Alternatively, if it is a question better fielded by a different provider, encourage the patient to ask that provider or reach out to the provider yourself and ask that person to contact the patient.

Testing a Fetus for Adult-Onset Conditions

Although not commonly pursued, occasionally a patient with a known diagnosis of an adult-onset condition will request a prenatal diagnostic testing to evaluate a fetus for that condition. With an increase in the availability of genetic testing, more and more genes are being identified for adult-onset conditions that may or may not have presymptomatic interventions or treatments available. If treatments are available, they may not be initiated until later in life. The option of testing a fetus for an adult-onset condition therefore raises specific issues that should be considered. It is the position of the NSGC to both support the patient's reproductive rights to make choices and to protect the rights of a minor. In testing of a minor, the NSGC recommends deferring testing if the results will not impact the medical management of or benefit the child. Because a fetus will most likely become a child, testing is therefore categorized as testing a minor. This violates the child's right and opportunity to decide on testing or not when he or she becomes an adult. Therefore, it is recommended that testing for adult-onset conditions in a fetus be deferred unless the management of the pregnancy would be affected. (Hercher et al., 2016). For example, a couple curious to know if their fetus has inherited the familial *BRCA* mutation should be encouraged to defer this testing. Alternatively, a patient with Huntington disease who would terminate an affected pregnancy may benefit from prenatal diagnosis.

Barriers for Consent

Providing informed consent is a cornerstone in the practice of genetic counseling. It is a key component of shared decision-making when it comes to a patient's health care. In this process, the provider has the goal to inform the patient of all the risks, benefits, limitations, uncertainties, and alternatives to the treatment, test, or procedure being presented. The patient, in turn, must have the competence to understand the provided information and the subsequent consequences of a decision and to authorize a choice voluntarily. All of the components of sharing complete information, patient understanding, and voluntary authorization need to be met for the consent process to be truly informed (Cordasco, 2013).

Although medical providers have a duty to uphold their part and provide accurate and complete information, occasionally informed consent will be compromised because patients either lack understanding or are not making a decision freely.

Patient Understanding

Common barriers that may be encountered in regards to patient understanding are patients who have intellectual disability or who speak a foreign language. Even patients who do not have these specific considerations may have a difficult time comprehending all the information and implications presented. A health care provider can help optimize the patient's understanding by providing information in the preferred language of the patient through the use of interpreters, repeating information, using visuals, and providing written documentation. For written information, organizations including the American Medical Association (Weiss, 2003) and National Institutes of Health (2017) recommend that the readability of patient information material should be no higher than a sixth-grade level. Providers can ask that the patient state in his or her own words what was discussed to assess understanding and then make any corrections if needed.

Voluntary Participation

Informed consent may also be influenced when the patient is not free to make a decision voluntarily. A common example is the treatment of a minor. A minor may present with a parent or be alone or with his or her significant other. Although a minor may benefit from parental involvement, there are times when the possibility of being influenced in a decision, may wish to make a decision about a pregnancy privately, or may be legally required to involve a personal representative (parent, guardian, or person *in loco parentis*) prior to making a decision. This raises the question of who is legally allowed to consent and who is allowed access to a minor's protected health information. Privacy provisions of the

Health Insurance Portability and Accountability Act (HIPAA) of 1996 allow a minor's personal representative to access the minor's records unless the minor is legally allowed to consent for that treatment or procedure. Most state statutes give minors the right to consent to treatment in specific situations which, depending on the state, may include treatment for prenatal care. This, however, may or may not include the option of termination; instead, many states require either parental notification and/or consent (National District Attorneys Association [NDAA], 2013).

Patients may also be heavily influenced into a decision by others. A situation sometimes encountered is a patient electing testing because she believes her "doctor wants her to." Perhaps the patient wants to please her doctor by being compliant, and she may be afraid to "disappoint" her provider. Perhaps the patient misinterpreted the provider's offering an option as a recommendation. Alternatively, it may be that she feels her doctor knows best and values professional direction regarding the decision. Although statements to respect a patient's rights are often directed toward health care providers, family members may also act to coerce, persuade, or manipulate a patient and her decision. It is important to recognize that, during the process of making a decision, many people will value and wish for their families' opinions; however, there are times in which a patient will choose an option against her will simply to accommodate others. When discussing options with patients, one should be mindful of different relationship dynamics and advocate for the patient by acknowledging that she alone has the right to make decisions regarding her care, even when her decisions contradict others' recommendations or preferences.

Rapidly Evolving Technologies

New developments in genetic testing technology and applications are occurring at an unprecedented pace. This is seen in all aspects of genetic testing and includes testing in the area of perinatal care. The introduction and adoption of new technologies into clinical practice can dramatically change current practices. The potential for change has been recently demonstrated with the availability of cfDNA testing for aneuploidy, expanded carrier testing, and microarray analysis for testing samples collected from diagnostic testing procedures. Now, with emerging options of cfDNA screening to test for single-gene conditions, cfDNA whole-genome analysis, and whole-exome sequencing possibilities, new changes to clinical practice may be around the corner. It is imperative for the health care provider to stay educated and up to date on new technologies and published guidelines.

Although significant research on the utility, risks, benefits, and limitations of any testing option should be fully evaluated before the option is integrated into clinical practice, many tests become clinically available before enough information is known. Just because a test becomes available does not make it an appropriate test. Additionally, although a certain method may be appropriate for testing in one clinical setting, such as pediatrics, it may not be appropriate to offer this testing for a fetus. If patients or other health care providers request additional information or the use of these tests on a pregnancy, the perinatal genetic counselor will have to navigate through the various options, review guidelines, and choose which tests their clinic will provide and which options will not be offered. The perinatal genetic counselor may have to tell a patient or other provider "no" when it comes to testing a fetus with a new test for various reasons (e.g., it has limited clinical utility) and be prepared to explain the reasoning behind those decisions. Additionally, a perinatal genetic counselor may be expected to be an "expert" in the field of genetics in their clinic, be up to date on all newly emerging technology, and provide advice on a test's potential use.

Conclusion

No one ever said genetic counseling is an easy profession. Not only is the information technical, complicated, and expanding at an unprecedented rate, but the social, legal, and ethical implications of working with patients and their families can be complex. This chapter highlights challenging situations that may be encountered in the perinatal setting. It is our hope that introducing these situations now will provide the reader with time to contemplate and self-reflect about possible responses to difficult situations in the future. Although these aspects of genetic counseling are difficult, they also present unique counseling opportunities, making this profession an extremely worthy and rewarding one.

References

American College of Obstetricians and Gynecologists Committee on Genetics. Committee Opinion no. 581: The use of chromosomal microarray analysis in prenatal diagnosis. *Obstet Gynecol.* 2013 Dec;122(6):1374–1377.

Bittles AH, Black ML. Consanguinity, human evolution, and complex diseases. *Proc Natl Acad Sci USA.* 2010;107(Suppl 1):1779–1786.

Cordasco KM. Obtaining informed consent from patients: brief update. Review. In: Making health care safer II: an updated critical analysis of the evidence for patient safety practices. Rockville, MD: Agency for Healthcare Research and Quality; 2013 Mar. (Evidence Reports/Technology Assessments, no. 211.) Chapter 39. https://www.ncbi.nlm.nih.gov/books/NBK133402/.

Cowley C. Conscientious objection in healthcare and the duty to refer. *J Med Ethics.* 2017 Apr;43(4):207–212. doi: 10.1136/medethics-2016-103928.

Crandall BF, Lebherz TB, Rubinstein L, Robertson RD, Sample WF, Sarti D, Howard J. Chromosome findings in 2,500 second trimester amniocenteses. *Am J Med Genet.* 1980;5(4):345–356.

Hercher L, Uhlmann WR, Hoffman EP. Prenatal testing for adult-onset conditions: the position of the National Society of Genetic Counselors. *J Genet Counsel.* 2016;25:1139.

Kearney HM, Thorland EC, Brown KK, Quintero-Rivera F, South ST. American College of Medical Genetics standards and guidelines for interpretation and reporting of postnatal constitutional copy number variants. *Genet Med.* 2011;13:680–685.

Maaji SM, Ekele BA, Bello SO, Morhason-Bello IO. Do women want disclosure of fetal gender during prenatal ultrasound scan? *Ann Afr Med.* 2010 Jan-Mar;9(1):11–14.

Muller C, Cameron LD. It's complicated—factors predicting decisional conflict in prenatal diagnostic testing. *Health Expect.* 2016;19(2):388–402.

National District Attorneys Association. Minor consent to treatment laws. http://www.ndaa.org/pdf/Minor%20Consent%20to%20 Medical%20Treatment%20(2).pdf. Published January, 2013. May 2017.

National Institutes of Health. How to write easy to read health materials. National Library of Medicine Web site. http://www. nlm.nih.gov/medlineplus/etr.html. Accessed Jun 2017.

Nielsen J, Wohlert M. Chromosome abnormalities found among 34,910 newborn children: results from a 13-year incidence study in Arhus, Denmark. *Hum Genet.* 1991 May;87(1):81–83.

Rehder CW, David KL, Hirsch B, Toriello HV, Wilson CM, Kearney HM. American College of Medical Genetics and Genomics: standards and guidelines for documenting suspected consanguinity as an incidental finding of genomic testing. *Genet Med.* 2013 Feb;15(2):150–152.

Shukar-Ud-Din S, Ubaid F, Shahani E, Saleh F. Reasons for disclosure of gender to pregnant women during prenatal ultrasonography. *Int J Womens Health.* 2013 Dec 13;5:781–785.

Tozzo P, Caenazzo L, Parker MJ. Discovering misattributed paternity in genetic counselling: different ethical perspectives in two countries. *J Med Ethics.* 2014 Mar;40(3):177–181.

US Department of Health and Human Services. The Surgeon General Family History Health Initiative. https://www.hhs. gov/programs/prevention-and-wellness/family-health-history/ index.html. Published 2004. May 2017.

Weiss BD. *Health literacy: a manual for clinicians.* Chicago, IL: American Medical Association, American Medical Foundation; 2003.

Westerfield L, Darilek S, van den Veyver IB. Counseling challenges with variants of uncertain significance and incidental findings in prenatal genetic screening and diagnosis. *J Clin Med.* 2014;3(3):1018–1032.

Wiseman M, Dancyger C, Michie S. Communicating genetic risk information within families: a review. *Fam Cancer.* 2010 Dec;9(4):691–703.

Voracek M, Haubner T, Fisher ML. Recent decline in nonpaternity rates: a cross-temporal meta-analysis. *Psychol Rep.* 2008 Dec;103(3):799–811.

Appendix A

Guidelines

The National Society of Genetic Counselors (NSGC), Society for Maternal–Fetal Medicine (SMFM), American College of Obstetricians and Gynecologists (ACOG), International Society of Prenatal Diagnosis (ISPD), American College of Medical Genetics and Genomics (ACMG), and American Society of Human Genetics (ASHG) have developed practice guidelines or committee opinions on the various testing options. Given guidelines change frequently, so it is recommended that the counselor visit these professional organizations for the most current recommendations. Here is list of professional organizations and their website information:

- National Society of Genetic Counselors www.nsgc.org
- American Congress of Obstetricians and Gynecologists www.acog.org
- Society for Maternal Fetal Medicine www.smfm.org
- American College of Medical Genetics and Genomics www.acmg.net
- International Society of Prenatal Diagnosis www.ispdhome.org
- American Society of Human Genetics www.ashg.org

Appendix B

Suggested Activities

Instructors (and students) may find the following activity suggestions useful in demonstrating and practicing the topics presented in this book. Activities may be completed in class or assigned as homework to be discussed later.

Activity 1: Practice Using a Pregnancy Wheel

Note to instructor: Provide students with a variety of scenarios to practice using a pregnancy wheel. Have them determine the expected due date, the estimated day of conception, when the patient should return for her 18- to 20-week ultrasound, and the like. Be sure to include complex examples, such as a pregnancy achieved using in vitro fertilization (IVF) with a 5-day frozen embryo, a pregnancy occurring in a leap year, or when an estimated delivery date (EDD) was based on ultrasound.

Example: A patient reports a last menstrual period (LMP) of April 14. What is the EDD?

Answer: January 19.

Activity 2: Determine Best EDD with Dating Discrepancies

Note to instructor: Have students practice case examples in which the patient's LMP does not match dating done by ultrasound. Present scenarios where the due date should be changed and ones where the due date should not be changed based on the available information.

Example: A patient reports an LMP of May 4. An ultrasound completed on July 23 reports the fetus is measuring 10 weeks 2 days. Based on this information, should the EDD be changed, and what EDD should be used?

Answer: No; February 23.

Activity 3: Practice G's and P's

Note to instructor: Give students a number of different pregnancy histories and have them write out G's and P's. Make sure to include complicated scenarios such as multiple pregnancies, premature births, ectopic pregnancies, and the like.

Example: A patient is currently in her third pregnancy. Her first pregnancy resulted in a miscarriage. The second pregnancy was twins, born at 36 weeks' gestation, but one was stillborn. What are her G's and P's?

Answer: G3P0111.

Activity 4: Take a Perinatal Medical and Family History

Note to instructor: Have students take mock pregnancy and family histories together or with friends. Alternatively, provide case examples for students to practice with. If providing case examples, include complex family history situations including family history of a genetic condition, twin pregnancies, consanguinity, same-sex couples, pregnancy losses (stillbirth and miscarriage), multiple reproductive partners, adoption, multifactorial conditions, and the like.

Example: A 28-year-old G3P1011 woman presents with a current pregnancy achieved by intrauterine implantation (IUI) using a sperm donor. She had a both a miscarriage at 8 weeks and a healthy son from a previous union. She has a family history of cystic fibrosis in which her male maternal first cousin is affected.

Answer:

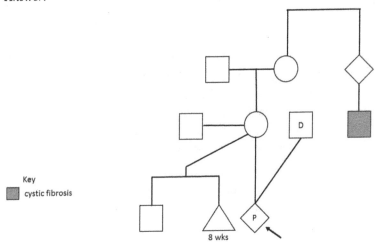

Key
cystic fibrosis

Activity 5: Determine Which Type of Testing to Offer Patients

Note to instructor: Provide a number of situations in which the student has to determine which testing option(s) should be offered. Students should be encouraged to use practice guidelines to determine the best course of action for an individual patient.

Example: A couple presents for preconception genetic counseling. The couple reports that they are both of Ashkenazi Jewish ancestry. What testing options should be offered?

Answer: Carrier testing for conditions more commonly seen in people with Ashkenazi Jewish ancestry cystic fibrosis spinal muscular atrophy (SMA), and consideration of expanded carrier testing.

Activity 6: Interpret Result Reports

Note to instructor: Give students a variety of result reports to interpret. Include examples of maternal serum screening, cell-free DNA (cfDNA), chromosome analysis, carrier testing, and more. Have examples that are within normal limits, abnormal, have incidental findings, or were ordered with incorrect information that needs updating. Have students interpret and discuss how they would manage the results and communicate the information to the patient.

Example: Provide an example of a quad screen with a high risk of Down syndrome. Also provide the students with an ultrasound report showing that the gestational age was overestimated by 15 days and changed. Therefore, the gestational age used on the quad screen was incorrect.

Answer: The student should explain that an overestimated gestational age can be a source for incorrect results on the quad screen and therefore should be recalculated.

Activity 7: Practice Determining and Discussing Sensitivity, Specificity, PPV, NPV

Note to instructor: Provide students with case examples in which they have to determine, calculate, or use online tools to calculate sensitivity, specificity, positive predictive value (PPV), and negative predictive value (NPV). Have students role-play the results. Emphasize the importance of practicing these discussions in patient-friendly language.

Example: A patient completed cfDNA testing with normal results. The patient is 40 years old. She is currently 12 weeks pregnant. The testing she completed has a sensitivity of 99% and specificity of 99%

for Down syndrome. The patient asks how likely it is that her baby has Down syndrome.

Answer: The student should calculate the NPV by a Bayesian analysis or by using an online tool (www.perinatalquality.org/vendors/nsgc/ nipt/) and communicate this to the patient.

Activity 8: Identify Testing Available and Logistics Required

Note to instructor: Have students research the testing available and the logistics required for prenatal diagnosis of a condition. Have students report which laboratory they selected, test turnaround time, sample requirements, paperwork needed, and the like.

Example: A patient is being seen because she is a known carrier of a premutation (56 repeats) in the *FMR1* gene associated with fragile-X. The pregnancy is currently of 16 weeks' gestation, and the fetus is male. The patient wishes to complete an amniocentesis. What is involved in ordering this test?

Answer: Students may use resources such as the genetic testing registry (https://www.ncbi.nlm.nih.gov/gtr/) to assist them in this activity. Answers will vary depending on the condition and the laboratory selected.

Activity 9: Present on an Ultrasound Anomaly and Its Implications

Note to instructor: Give each student an assigned ultrasound finding .) and have each student develop a presentation and teach each other. Required topics to include in the presentation are an overview of the embryology, how the condition is diagnosed (including ultrasound features), differential diagnosis, clinical importance, mode of inheritance, genetic counseling issues, management issues affecting both the pregnancy and the neonate, and prenatal genetic testing (availability of genetic testing, technology used, available labs, timing of testing, etc.).

Example: Ultrasound findings could include cystic hygroma, rhabdomyoma, omphalocele, ambiguous genetalia, etc.

Answer: Answers will vary depending on the condition assigned.

Activity 10: Discuss the Use of a Medication with a Patient During Pregnancy

Note to instructor: Have students research an assigned medication. Suggest that they use resources such as Reprotox or other available resources including books, published articles, and call centers. Have students role-play discussing the use of the medication during pregnancy, including pros, cons, testing options, registries, and the like. Use both known teratogens (e.g., uncontrolled diabetes, valproic acid, and oral isotretinoin) and medications known to be safe in pregnancy. Alternatively, role-playing students can present their assigned medication in class with a short formal or informal presentation.

Example: A patient is taking Lamictal to treat her personal history of epilepsy.

Answer: Students should discuss the possibility of an increased risk of an oral cleft after exposure to Lamictal during pregnancy but also mention how studies have been inconsistent with this finding. A recommendation of an 18- to 20-week ultrasound with special attention to the fetal face should be recommended. Also, the patient should be encouraged to contact the Antiepileptic Drug Pregnancy Registry and provide more information about a teratogen risk line.

Activity 11: With a Partner, Discuss Termination as a Pregnancy Management Option

Note to instructor: Have students role-play or do a group discussion about how they would offer the option of pregnancy termination to patients and discuss the actual process, including legal implications, risks, alternatives, procedure options, and support available. Provide them with case examples of people with a variety of different findings including both lethal and nonlethal anomalies (anencephaly vs. Down syndrome), varying gestational ages (first vs second trimester), and more complex situations (twins, late-term).

Example: An ultrasound identifies anencephaly in a fetus at 20 weeks' gestation.

Answer: The student should discuss available options to continue the pregnancy or to complete a pregnancy termination for a lethal anomaly. Legal implications, resources, and referrals will vary depending on state.

Activity 12: Observations for Further Learning

Note to instructor: Provide the students with a variety of different procedure or clinic observation options depending on their availability in local clinics.

Example: Observations could include ultrasound examinations, diagnostic testing procedures (amniocentesis or chorionic villus sampling, fetal echocardiogram), autopsy, fetal magnetic resonance imaging, embryo transfer, shadowing at Planned Parenthood for a day, shadowing or attending a perinatal hospice or support group, and the like.

Answer: Have the student provide their thoughts and feelings about observing the procedures or clinics. Can be in writing or as a verbal discussion.

Activity 13: Research and Present on Available Supplemental Support and Referral Options

Note to instructor: Provide students with a variety of case examples and have them research support and referral options that they would recommend or offer to a patient. Case examples could include situations for students to suggest support groups (e.g., Cystic Fibrosis Foundation), adoption options for a pregnancy affected with Down syndrome, couple counseling services, social work referrals (patient reports domestic violence during session), and other providers (cardiologist).

Example: A patient states that she is having a hard time dealing with the loss of her prior child who was affected with SMA. She asks if there are any counselors who specialize in grief counseling that you could recommend.

Answer: Answers will vary depending on local support options but could include counselors in the area who provide grief counseling or SMA support groups.

Activity 14: Discuss Complex Counseling Situations

Note to instructor: Provide students with a complex counseling scenario. The students should discuss how they think they would respond to the person or couple and why they chose this response.

Example: You are counseling a 38-year-old primigravid woman and her 40-year-old husband for advanced maternal age. The pregnancy has completed 16.4 weeks of gestation by dates. A 9-week viability check was done in the referring doctor's office. An ultrasound examination for fetal anatomy and amniocentesis, should the couple elect to pursue it, is scheduled immediately after the genetic counseling. The couple's family history is unremarkable. The couple is conflicted about whether to pursue amniocentesis. The man asks you, "What would you do in our situation?"

Example: A 22-year-old primigravid woman and her 25-year-old partner see you for genetic counseling because of an abnormal maternal serum screen. The Down syndrome risk is 1 in 27. The woman is leaning toward pursuing amniocentesis. When you ask her partner for his opinion about whether they should do amniocentesis, he replies, "It's her body, so it's up to her."

Answer: For each scenario, there will likely not be one "correct" answer (unless it is a blatant violation of the Code of Ethics).

Index

Tables and figures are indicated by an italic *t* and *f* following the page/paragraph number.